Handbook of
Phlebotomy
and Patient Service
Techniques

FOURTH EDITION

Handbook of
Phlebotomy
and Patient Service Techniques

F O U R T H   E D I T I O N

Garland E. Pendergraph, Ph.D., SM(ASCP)
Director of Education and Satellite Laboratory Director
Doctors Laboratory, Inc.
Valdosta, Georgia

Cynthia Barfield Pendergraph, MT(ASCP)
Laboratory/X-Ray Manager
Tifton Physicians Center
Tifton, Georgia

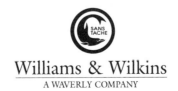

Williams & Wilkins
A WAVERLY COMPANY

BALTIMORE • PHILADELPHIA • LONDON • PARIS • BANGKOK
BUENOS AIRES • HONG KONG • MUNICH • SYDNEY • TOKYO • WROCLAW

Editor: Donna Balado
Managing Editor: Jennifer Schmidt
Marketing Manager: Peter Darcy
Project Editor: Ulita Lushnycky
Design Coordinator: Mario Fernandez

Copyright © 1998 Williams & Wilkins

351 West Camden Street
Baltimore, Maryland 21201-2436 USA

Rose Tree Corporate Center
1400 North Providence Road
Building II, Suite 5025
Media, Pennsylvania 19063-2043 USA

The publisher is not responsible (as a matter of product liability, negligence or otherwise) for any injury resulting from any material contained herein. This publication contains information relating to general principles of medical care which should not be construed as specific instructions for individual patients. Manufacturers' product information and package inserts should be reviewed for current information, including contraindications, dosages and precautions.

Printed in the United States of America

First Edition, 1984
Reprinted, 1985, 1987
Second Edition, 1988
Reprinted, 1989, 1990, 1991
Third Edition, 1992
Reprinted, 1993, 1994, 1996
Fourth Edition, 1998

Library of Congress Cataloging-in-Publication Data

Pendergraph, Garland E.
    Handbook of phlebotomy and patient service techniques / Garland E. Pendergraph, Cynthia Barfield Pendergraph. — 4th ed.
      p.   c.m.
    Rev. ed. of: handbook of phlebotomy. 3rd ed. 1992.
    Includes bibliographical references and index.
    ISBN 0-683-30556-5 (pbk.)
    1. Phlebotomy—Handbooks, manuals, etc. I. Pendergraph, Cynthia Barfield. II. Pendergraph, Garland E. Handbook of phlebotomy. III. Title.
    [DNLM: 1. Phlebotomy—methods handbooks. WB 39 P397h 1998]
    RB45.15.P46 1998
    616.07′561—dc21
    DNLM/DLC
    for Library of Congress   98-13761
                                    CIP

The publishers have made every effort to trace the copyright holders for borrowed material. If they have inadvertently overlooked any, they will be pleased to make the necessary arrangements at the first opportunity.

To purchase additional copies of this book, call our customer service department at **(800) 638-0672** or fax orders to **(800) 447-8438.** For other book services, including chapter reprints and large quantity sales, ask for the Special Sales department.

Canadian customers should call **(800) 665-1148,** or fax **(800) 665-0103.** For all other calls originating outside of the United States, please call **(410) 528-4223** or fax us at **(410) 528-8550.**

Visit Williams & Wilkins on the Internet: http://www.wwilkins.com or contact our customer service department at **custserv@wwilkins.com.** Williams & Wilkins customer service representatives are available from 8:30 am to 6:00 pm, EST, Monday through Friday, for telephone access.

98 99 00 01 02
1 2 3 4 5 6 7 8 9 10

To the laboratory's envoys to the outside world:
the phlebotomists
and
To the employees of Doctors Laboratory, Inc.,
who have made my life so enjoyable
and my work such a pleasure.

Preface

Although the approach of this new edition remains the same as previous ones, the changes are numerous—noticeably in the area of safety and infection prevention. Added too are new procedures and concepts that may be used as phlebotomists assume new health care roles. It is important for the reader to be cognizant of the fact, however, that there is more than one correct method or system application. Equally important to understand is that this book in no way pretends to be a definitive work on the subject of phlebotomy or patient service techniques. Students are advised to search out a variety of resources in their studies.

There are many to whom I am eternally grateful. First, I wish to express my appreciation to those individuals who helped me with the previous three editions. Without their cooperation and encouragement, this fourth edition would never have been. I wish to thank Bill McGehee MT(ASCP), Monika Patel, MT(ASCP), Linda Cason, MT(HEW), Steve Siebert, and Sean Henry who generously let us use them as our models in several of the photographs and to C. D. Richards, DVM, and his associates who graciously gave of their time to assist in making the veterinary pictures. My appreciation to those companies that allowed me to illustrate their products and to the staff of Williams and Wilkins who gently prodded me on when I became slack. Also, a special thank you to those who offered suggestions and constructive criticism regarding the previous editions. I am most appreciative to Fran Delaney who, in spite of my indecisions and many revisions, patiently took the photographs used in this edition. Last but not least, I am greatly indebted to my coauthor who not only helped write portions of this fourth edition, but scrupulously edited each chapter for oversights.

Finally, I remember that a friend once philosophized to me that those who would be able to survive into the 21st century would be those who could rapidly adapt to change. As the millennium quickly comes to a close, I tend to reflect on what he said more often. Certainly as we daily hear the need to cross-train or be multi-skilled and about consolidation and downsizing, one cannot help but be apprehensive about the future. Nonetheless, those individuals who display their competency through certification or licensure, actively participate in a professional organization, and enhance their skills through continuing education will be better prepared to survive into the 21st century than those who are satisfied with the status quo.

Garland E. Pendergraph
Cynthia Barfield Pendergraph

Contents

PROFESSIONAL
CONCERNS

A Brief History of
Phlebotomy

An interesting fact about the history of phlebotomy is the lack of history about phlebotomy insofar as the "letting" of blood for diagnostic rather than therapeutic purposes. The "letting" of blood for "healing" purposes has been practiced since antiquity, and practically every civilization has recorded its use. Phlebotomy was used as a therapeutic measure in the United States well into the eighteenth century.

Little is known about when blood was first used to diagnose disease. A bit more is known about the origin of the instruments of phlebotomy as they pertain to attaining blood for analysis. The familiar piston-and-cylinder syringe was first used on wounds as a "pus-puller." Its precise birth record is lost, but the concept of the piston and cylinder is attributed to the ingenuity of Ktesibios, the son of a barber in Alexandria, Egypt, around 280 BC. Its use to extract pus from wounds and another possible use—as a flame thrower—never caught on. This great instrument (an early example is illustrated in Figure 1.1) has been used during most of its existence for the injection of liquids.

The date when blood first began to be examined for diagnostic purposes is unknown, although it is known that another body fluid, urine, has been examined since medieval times. The invention of the microscope in the seventeenth century, coupled with advancements in physiologic chemistry and cellular physiology in the nineteenth century, paved the way for the examination of blood as a diagnostic tool probably in the latter part of the nineteenth century.

It was not until 1908 that the first Manual of Clinical Diagnosis was published. The author was James C. Todd, a professor of clinical pathology at the University of Colorado School of Medicine. A sentence that will amuse most laboratorians is located in the chapter "The Blood" in the 1912 edition. It reads: "For most clinical examinations only one drop of blood is required." The manual described general techniques for obtaining blood by venipuncture and skin stick and discussed the latest laboratory procedures. A few of the important ones included the cigarette-paper (Zig-zag brand) method for

3

FIGURE 1.1 An early piston-and-cylinder syringe. (Reprinted with permission from Majno G. The healing hand: man and wound in the ancient world. Cambridge: Harvard University Press, 1975.)

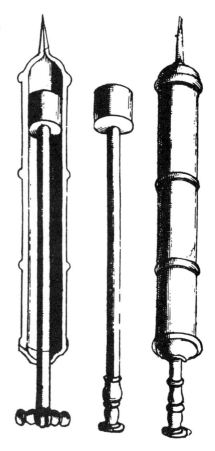

making differential slides; fixing differential slides before staining by soaking them in pure methyl alcohol for 15 minutes or heating them in an oven at 150°C; and obtaining a blood culture from a skin puncture in the lobe of the ear. "By gentle milking, 20 to 40 drops can usually be obtained."

A few of the instruments that were recommended in early editions for use in obtaining blood are illustrated in Figures 1.2, 1.3, and 1.4. Although the instrumentation recommended may appear somewhat crude as compared with the instrumentation of today, the concepts remain similar.

Little change occurred in either instrumentation or concepts until 1943 when an evacuated blood collection system, known as the VACUTAINER Brand, had its beginning. This system is discussed in more detail in Chapter 8. This was not the first evacuated system. The Keidel vacuum tube for the collection of blood was manufactured by Hynson, Wescott and Dunning (located in Baltimore, Maryland) in approximately 1922. This system consisted

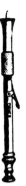

FIGURE 1.2 Army-type blood lancet. (Reprinted with permission from Todd JC, Sanford AH, Wells BB. Clinical diagnosis by laboratory methods, 12th ed. Philadelphia: WB Saunders, 1953.)

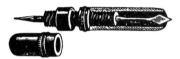

FIGURE 1.3 Daland's blood lancet. (Reprinted with permission from Todd JC. Clinical diagnosis by laboratory methods, 5th ed. Philadelphia: WB Saunders, 1923.)

FIGURE 1.4 A device for drawing blood from a vein using a large test tube. (Reprinted with permission from Todd JC: Clinical diagnosis by laboratory methods, 8th ed. Philadelphia: WB Saunders, 1937.)

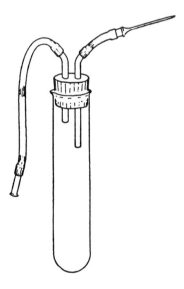

of a sealed ampule with or without culture medium. Connected to the ampule was a short rubber tube with a needle at the end (Fig. 1.5). A small glass tube served as a cap. After the needle had been inserted into the vein, the stem of the ampule was crushed. The blood entered the ampule because of the vacuum. This concept did not become popular until the introduction of the VACUTAINER Brand. I own a Keidel vacuum tube with culture medium that was manufactured in 1922. The culture medium is still sterile.

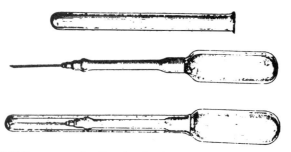

FIGURE 1.5 Keidel's vacuum tube. (Reprinted with permission from Todd JC: Clinical diagnosis by laboratory methods, 8th ed. Philadelphia: WB Saunders, 1937.)

The introduction of the VACUTAINER Brand and similar evacuated blood collection systems initiated a new interest in improving techniques and reconsidering concepts related to phlebotomy. Great strides have been made since the days of manually sharpened needles with their ever-present and painful "burrs." Not only are needles now smaller and sharper and skin lancets properly sterilized and less painful, but newer concepts of obtaining blood more effectively assure more accurate results and less permanent damage to the patient.

Today there are several national organizations (See *Appendix*) that administer certifying examinations for phlebotomists. The first, The National Phlebotomy Association (NPA), was founded in 1978. What the future holds for phlebotomy is unknown, but transition is certain. It can be said without fear of contradiction, however, that the numerous scientific improvements and changes in philosophy reflect the efforts and contributions of many individuals who realize that correctly obtaining a specimen for laboratory testing is more than just a "sideline" but rather a vital step in the early and proper diagnosis of disease.

No history of phlebotomy is complete without mentioning the history of circulation. The identity of the first person to recognize the importance of veins and arteries is lost with antiquity; however, as long ago as 2650 BC, Hwang-Ti, Emperor of China, made the observation that "all blood is under the control of the heart. The blood flows continuously in a circle and never stops." Even Hippocrates (460 to 375 BC), the father of medicine, noted: "The vessels spread themselves over the body filling it with spirit, juice, and motion are all of them but branches of an original vessel. I protest I know not where it begins or where it ends, for in a circle there is neither a beginning nor an end."

It would be another 2000 years before the correct movement of blood from the heart and its return to it would be outlined. Praxagoras of Cos (340 BC) was among the first to separate the functions of arteries and veins but believed that both systems contained air. It was Galen (AD 130 to 200) (Fig. 1.6), an egotistical Greek physician from Pergamon, who showed that arteries are filled with blood, not air, which was still the prevalent thinking of the time. Galen also showed, with fair accuracy, the heart movements. But he did not stop there; he went on to theorize that the blood moved from the right side of the heart to the left through pores in the walls between the ventricles. This theory was but one of his many anatomic mistakes.

That little or no knowledge was contributed about the circulation of blood for centuries after Galen's death testifies to his dictatorship over medicine until the critics of the Renaissance toppled him. For approximately the next 1500 years, men bowed to authority. Because the church had embraced the writings of Galen as the absolute truth, to propose other hypotheses contrary to Galen's teachings would be heresy. Many a man of science was slowly burned at the stake for doing so.

From time to time, there was a flicker of light. In approximately AD 1531, Michael Servetus maintained that the blood passed from one side of the heart to the other through the lungs. For his discovery of pulmonic circulation, he was rewarded by having his books confiscated and being burned at the stake.

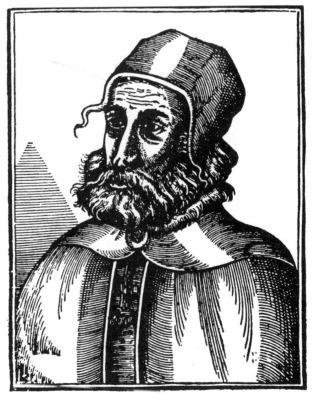

FIGURE 1.6 Galen, AD 130–200. (Reprinted with permission from Haggard HW. Devils, drugs and doctors. New York: Harper and Row, 1929.)

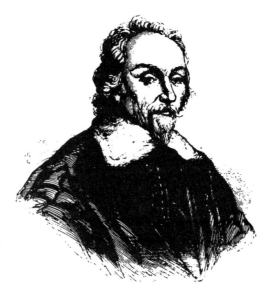

FIGURE 1.7   Harvey, AD 1578–1657. (Reprinted with permission from Russell JR. History and heroes of the art of medicine. London: John Murray, 1861.)

In AD 1628 in a lecture before the Fellows of the Royal College of Physicians, William Harvey (Fig. 1.7) followed the passage of blood from the heart, through the arteries, to the veins, and back to the heart again. It was as if Hwang-Ti, that Emperor of China, had been his mentor. Actually, it was his anatomy professor, Fabricius of Aquapendente, and his work on the valves of the veins that gave stimulus to Harvey's conclusions.

How the blood passed from the arteries into the veins remained a mystery until approximately AD 1660 when Marcello Malpighi, the leading microscopist of his time, demonstrated capillary circulation.

BIBLIOGRAPHY

1. Haggard HW. Devils, drugs and doctors. New York: Harper and Row, 1929.
2. Heath-Hammond LR, Gelinas CE. A history of phlebotomy in 18th-century America. Laboratory Medicine 1982;13:776.
3. Majno G. The healing hand: man and wound in the ancient world. Cambridge: Harvard University Press, 1975.
4. Neuburger M. History of medicine, vol 1. Oxford: Oxford University Press, 1910.
5. Poynter FNL, Keele KD. A short history of medicine. London: Mills and Boon, 1961.
6. Robinson V. The story of medicine. New York: Tudor Publishing, 1931.

7. Todd JC. Clinical diagnosis by laboratory methods, 2nd ed. Philadelphia: WB Saunders, 1912.
8. Todd JC. Clinical diagnosis by laboratory methods, 5th ed. Philadelphia: WB Saunders, 1923.
9. Todd JC, Sanford AH, Wells BB. Clinical diagnosis by laboratory methods, 12th ed. Philadelphia: WB Saunders, 1953.
10. Walker K. The story of blood. London: Herbert Jenkins, 1958.
11. Williams MR, Lindberg DS. An introduction to the profession of medical technology, 3rd ed. Philadelphia: Lea & Febiger, 1979.

Professionalism

The term *professional* seems to mean many different things to different people. A high school athlete may think of a professional as being a highly paid player who plays for a ranked sports team. To a stockbroker, the term is likely to bring to mind clients who are lawyers or physicians. The dictionary defines a professional as one who is "following an occupation as a means of livelihood or for gain." Current thought broadens the often used traditional definition that, historically, limited recognized professions to the learned disciplines of theology, law, or medicine. As technology has advanced and specialization at work has grown, other disciplines of learning are now considered as professions.

For our purposes, a professional is defined as an individual who performs his/her work with expertise, mastery, and skill. A professional is a person who has been extensively trained or disciplined to render a particular service and is governed by an organized body that regulates continued practice in this field by requiring (1) adherence to a code of ethics and (2) an assessment of competency.

The professionalism a health care worker displays by learning and correctly performing work in a health care field can be further enhanced by personal work habits that are displayed by health care workers while "on the job." How many times have you heard someone say, "That person is very unprofessional!"? Well, it could mean that the person was being loud and rude or just wearing a dirty lab coat. The aura of professionalism covers a very broad range of behaviors and the appearance of a health care worker.

In addition to honesty and confidentiality, another important aspect of professionalism is the health care worker's personal appearance. I recall a personal experience while shopping at a hardware store. The owner of the store asked whether I was acquainted with an individual who was employed at the local hospital. I indicated the name was familiar, but the person had resigned from the laboratory staff just before I had arrived as the laboratory director. The store owner commented, "I'm glad to hear he is no longer with you. The

12

Seen in the emergency room while he was on call, he came
...ad just finished feeding the pigs." In all probability, the
few ti...erious doubts about the results of the laboratory tests be-
in lo...ervations concerning the appearance of the person who came
stor...od.
cau
to ... dress and grooming are extremely important aspects of profes-
...arance, they are not the entire picture. Times are changing; but
...tive dress is still appropriate because many patients undergoing gen-
...lth care are older. Appearance instills confidence. Shirts that are worn
...t of a uniform should not display any emblem or logo except that of the
...th care institution. Uniforms or professional attire will be dictated by each
...alth care institution. Even so, attire should be clean and unwrinkled. Only
closed-toe, nonskid-sole shoes should be worn. Shoes should be as clean as
possible.

Hair should be clean, and long hair should be pulled away from the face
so that it will not fall forward when bending over patients. Beards and mus-
taches of staff members should be neatly trimmed. Otherwise, the face should
be shaved, not stubbled with 1- or 2-day hair growth.

Health care worker's hands must be clean. Fingernails should be groomed
and should not be so long that they hamper or interfere with providing health
care. Garish fingernail polish colors should be avoided because they are inappropriate to a health care setting. Body odor should be undetectable. Fresh
breath will be most appreciated, not only by patients, but also by fellow employees. Excessive jewelry should be avoided. Only wedding bands and class
rings should be worn on the hands. Long earrings are inappropriate (and possibly unsafe) to wear while on duty.

Like professionalism, ethics is also hard to define. Bissell and Cosman state
"ethics consists of far more than abiding by rules, procedures, and guidelines.
. . . Ethics represents what we should do, not what we must do. It represents
an expression of conscience. . . ." Health care workers who are professional
should not act as they might otherwise act away from their job. Rather, professional health care workers discipline themselves to take those actions that
are required under the circumstances to do the job the best way possible. Of
course, these actions need to adhere to the policies and procedures established
by the health care institution.

We have defined professional, but "acting professional" or "professionalism" is much more difficult to define because the meaning covers such a wide
range of activities. Most professional societies have a "code of ethics," a principle of right or good conduct. The code of ethics outlines what must and
must not be done in order to avoid harming the life, well-being, or privacy of
the recipient of that service. Laboratorians do not reveal the results of laboratory tests to anyone except authorized persons because to do so would vi-
olate a principle of good conduct. It would be unethical, thus, unprofessional.

A code of ethics defines the ethical behavior required of member employees. The following is an example of a code of ethics used by the associate members of the American Society of Clinical Pathologists (ASCP). It is as follows:

Recognizing that my integrity and that of my profession must be pledged to the best possible care of patients based on the reliability of my work, I will:

- Treat patients and colleagues with respect, care, and thoughtfulness
- Perform my duties in an accurate, precise, timely, and responsible manner
- Safeguard patient information as confidential, within the limits of the law
- Prudently use laboratory resources
- Advocate the delivery of quality laboratory services in a cost-effective manner
- Work within the boundaries of the laws and regulations and strive to disclose illegal or improper behavior to the appropriate authorities
- Continue to study, apply, and advance medical laboratory knowledge and skills and share such with my colleagues, other members of the health care community, and the public

Health care workers must be prepared to deal in a professional manner with patients and other health care workers. The health care worker who appears unhurried, who is considerate and gentle when handling patients, and who speaks in an authoritative but quiet voice further enhances the patient's confidence in that health care worker and in the results of health care work that is being performed.

BIBLIOGRAPHY

Becan-McBride K, ed: Textbook of clinical laboratory supervision. New York: Appleton-Century-Crofts, 1982.

Bissell M, Cosman T. How ethical dilemmas induce stress. Medical Laboratory Observer 1991;23:28.

College of American Pathologists. So you're going to collect a blood specimen. Skokie, IL: College of American Pathologists, 1974.

Williams MR, Lindberg DS. An introduction to the profession of medical technology, 3rd ed. Philadelphia: Lea & Febiger, 1979.

Medical Terminology and Abbreviations

Communication is an essential part of any job or profession; nowhere is good communication more important than in health-related fields. Communication is best when one uses terms that everyone can understand. Why say that someone has "pharyngitis" when all you are trying to convey is that the person has a "sore throat"? On the other hand, sometimes general terms do not adequately describe the problem. A severe sharp pain along the glossopharyngeal nerve causes a "sore throat." The term "glossopharyngeal neuralgia" better communicates what caused the "sore throat" and distinguishes it from other types of sore throats such as "strep throat," which is more familiar. In other words, in medicine, as in all other professions, certain terms give exact meanings that cannot be conveyed by simpler means. It is imperative, then, that all professionals in the medical field, not just physicians and nurses, be familiar with the most frequently used medical terminology.

This section is divided into four parts. The first part gives important prefixes, suffixes, and word roots, which, even if you do not know the definition of medical terms, will give you a clue to some of their meanings. The second part is a list of words or terms that should be in the vocabulary of any health care worker. The third part is a list of often used abbreviations and symbols. The last section contains the names of commonly ordered laboratory tests and their basic clinical usefulness.

It would be negligent to end the introduction of this section without mentioning that communication is a two-way street. *Listening is just as important as talking.*

PREFIXES, SUFFIXES, AND WORD ROOTS

Word Part	Meaning	Example
a, an	without	*a*pnea
aer/o	air	*aer*obic
algia	pain	neur*algia*
angi/o	vessel	*angi*ospasm
anti	against	*anti*biotics
arthr	joint	*arth*
bi	two	*bi*focal
bio	life	*bio*logy
blast	embryonic cell	myelo*blast*
brady	slow	*brady*cardia
calci	stone	*calc*
card	heart	*card*iac
ceph	head	en*ceph*alitis
cerebr	skull	*cerebr*um
cut	skin	sub*cut*aneous
cyst	bladder, hollow	*cyst*otomy
cyte	cell	leuko*cyte*
dent	tooth	*dent*ist
derm	skin	epi*derm*is
di	through	*di*gestion
dipl	double	*dipl*ococcus
dys	difficult	*dys*menorrhea
ectomy	removal	gastr*ectomy*
emesis	vomiting	hyper*emesis*
emia	blood	an*emia*
end	within	*end*ocardium
epi	on, upon	*epi*dermis
erythr	red	*erythr*ocyte
gast	stomach	*gast*rectomy
geri	old age	*geri*atrics
glyc	sweet	*glyc*ogen
gyne	woman	*gyne*cology
hem	blood	*hem*atology
hepat	liver	*hepat*ic
hist	tissue	*hist*ology
hydr	water	*hydr*ophobia
hyper	above normal	*hyper*thyroidism
hypo	below normal	*hypo*glycemia
hyster	uterus	*hyster*ectomy

Word Part	Meaning	Example
inter	between	*inter*stitial
intra	within	*intra*cellular
itis	inflammation	dermat*itis*
leuk	white	*leuk*emia
lysis	breakdown	hemo*lysis*
macr/o	large	*macr*ocyte
mal	bad	*mal*ignancy
meg	great, large	hepato*meg*aly
men	menses	*men*struation
mening	meninges	*mening*itis
micr	small	*micr*obe
morph	form	*morph*ology
myo	muscle	*myo*cardium
neph	kidney	*neph*ritis
neur	nerve	*neur*ology
noso	relating to disease	*noso*comial
oma	tumor	melan*oma*
onc	tumor, mass	*onc*ology
orrhea	flow or discharge	py*orrhea*
orth	straight, correct	*orth*ostatic
os, oste	bone	*oste*omyelitis
osis	condition	sarcoid*osis*
otomy	incision	duoden*otomy*
par	to give birth to	post*par*tum
para	beside, near	*para*thyroid
path	sick	*path*ogenic
penia	decrease in	leuko*penia*
peri	around	*peri*cardium
phleb	vein	*phleb*otomy
pneum	air	*pneum*onia
poly	many	*poly*cythemia
post	behind (position)	*post*nasal
post	after (time)	*post*partum
pre	in front of (position)	*pre*hyoid
pre	before (time)	*pre*natal
psych	mind	*psych*osis
pulm	lung	*pulm*onary
py, pyr	fever, heat	*pyr*exia
pyel	renal	*pyel*onephritis
rhin	nose	*rhin*orrhea

Word Part	Meaning	Example
salping	fallopian tube	*salping*itis
sanguin	bloody	*sanguin*al
scler	hard	*scler*otic
stasis	act or condition of stopping	hemo*stasis*
sub	below, under	*sub*acute
tach	rapid	*tach*ycardia
thromb	clot	*thromb*osis
tox	poison	anti*tox*in
tri	three	*tri*cuspid
ven	vein	*ven*esection

WORDS AND TERMS

Word/Term	Meaning
Accessioning	the first step in processing a specimen, when you give it a specific number or code
Accuracy	as near to the real answer as possible
Acrocyanosis	a blueness of the hands or feet caused by disturbances to the superficial veins
Adenoma	a tumor of glandular superficial epithelium
Aerobic	lives in the presence of oxygen
Allergy	an abnormal (hypersensitive) reaction to an agent or condition
Anaerobic	able to live without oxygen
Anastomosis	a communication between two vessels, either end to end or by means of a connecting channel
Anemia	deficiency of red blood cells, hemoglobin, or both
Aneurysm	a bulge in an artery caused by a weakening of its wall
Anorexia	loss of appetite
Antibiotic	a substance used in the treatment of infectious diseases, usually caused by bacteria

Word/Term	Meaning
Antibody	a protective body protein produced as a result of exposure to an antigen
Anticoagulant	a substance that delays or prevents the blood from clotting
Antigen	a substance that stimulates a specific resistance response and thus causes the body to produce antibodies
Antimicrobial	a substance that either kills or inhibits microscopic organisms
Apnea	a temporary cessation of breathing
Arteriosclerosis	hardening of the arteries
Asepsis	free from germs or infection
Bacteria	one-cell microscopic organisms that either cause disease (pathogenic) or do not cause disease (non-pathogenic); many different kinds of bacteria normally live on the skin and in the intestine, and are referred to as "normal flora"
Bacteriology	the study of bacteria
Bacteriostatic	inhibits, but does not kill bacteria
Bradycardia	slow heartbeat
Carcinogenic	anything that is capable of or conducive to the production of cancer
Carcinoma	a malignant tumor (cancer)
Cardiology	that branch of medicine that deals with heart disease
Cardiovascular	pertaining to the heart and blood vessels
Carrier	a person who is able to spread to others a disease with which he is infected but of which he usually has no symptoms
Centrifuge	a piece of laboratory equipment that spins test tubes at high speed and separates the cellular and liquid portions of the blood

Word/Term	Meaning
Cephalgia	headache
Clot	coagulated blood
Coagulate	to change from a fluid state into a semisolid mass
Coccus	a type of bacterium that is spherical in form
Collateral	side by side, subordinate
Communicable	refers to a disease that may be spread either directly or indirectly from one person to another
Coumadin	an anticoagulant or blood-thinning agent also known as warfarin; prothrombin time determinations are essential for its proper control
Crenated	notched red blood cells
Croup	a childhood disease that is characterized by a barking cough and difficult breathing
Cyanosis	a condition in which the skin turns a bluish color because of lack of oxygen to the blood
Cystic fibrosis	an inherited disorder of the exocrine glands that causes them to produce thick secretions of mucus; obstruction of the small bowel and persistent upper respiratory infections may result
Cystitis	inflammation of the urinary bladder
Differential	a percentage of each type of white blood cell in a total of 100 white cells observed
Digoxin	a drug used to strengthen heart contractions, also known as Lanoxin
Disinfect	to kill disease-causing germs
Dysentery	a diarrhea in which blood or mucus or both may be present in the feces
Dyspnea	difficulty in breathing
Ectopic	away from or out of the normal location

Word/Term	Meaning
Edema	a condition in which the body tissues contain an excessive amount of fluid, resulting in swelling
Embolus	a blood clot or some other mass (which may be solid, liquid, or gaseous) that stops up a blood vessel, brought to the plugged vessel from another area
Emphysema	a chronic disease of the lungs in which there is an improper exchange of oxygen and carbon dioxide
Empyema	pus in a body cavity, especially in the chest cavity
Encephalitis	inflammation of the brain
Endocarditis	inflammation of the inner lining of the heart, including the heart valves
Endocrine	pertains to a group of ductless glands that secrete a substance or hormone into the bloodstream or affect other organs directly
Endocrinology	branch of medicine that deals with diseases of the ductless glands (e.g., pituitary or thyroid glands)
Endogenous	something produced within a cell or organism
Endothelium	a layer of flat cells that lines the inner surface of the entire circulatory system
Enteric	pertaining to the intestinal tract
Enzyme	a complex compound that is able to initiate chemical changes in the body
Epithelium	a layer of cells that covers the internal and external surfaces of the body
Exocrine	secretion through a narrow tubular structure (duct) that opens onto an organ, tissue, or vessel
Exogenous	something produced outside a cell or organism (e.g., endogenous obesity would be caused by a dysfunction of the metabolic systems, whereas exogenous obesity would be caused by eating too many high-calorie foods)

Word/Term	Meaning
Exudate	fluid secreted by tissue, which may occur normally, but is usually in response to inflammation, damage, or irritation
Febrile	with fever
Fibrillation	quivering of the heart muscle rather than normal contraction
Fistula	an abnormal tube-like canal extending from one organ to another
Gastralgia	stomachache
Gastritis	inflammation of the lining of the stomach
Gastroenterology	branch of medicine concerned with the physiology and pathology of the stomach, intestines, and related areas
Gastrointestinal	having to do with the stomach and intestines
Gauge	as used in the laboratory, a unit of measurement determining the dimension of a needle
Geriatric	that branch of medicine that deals with the health and diseases of the elderly
Germicide	a substance that kills germs
Glomerulonephritis	inflammation of the filtering units of the kidneys
Gram's stain	a special stain used to help classify bacteria into two groups: gram-positive and gram-negative
Gynecology	branch of medicine that deals with diseases of the female reproductive organs
Hematocrit	a laboratory test in which the red blood cells are centrifuged at a high speed so they will be separated from blood serum and their volume can be expressed as a percentage of the total volume
Hematology	study of blood and its diseases
Hematoma	a mass of blood that is collected in the tissue and is caused by a break in a blood vessel

Word/Term	Meaning
Hemoconcentration	a rapid increase in the relative red blood cell content in the blood
Hemolysis	destruction of the red blood cells
Hemophilia	a hereditary disease characterized by a prolonged clotting time of the blood
Hemorrhage	abnormal internal or external bleeding
Hepatic	having to do with the liver
Hepatitis	inflammation of the liver usually resulting from an infection by a transmissible virus
Hepatomegaly	enlarged liver
Hormone	a substance that is produced by a ductless gland and is carried to other parts of the body by the blood; it exerts control over many of the body's processes
Host	a plant or animal in which a parasite lives
Hyperglycemia	excessive amount of sugar in the blood
Hyperkalemia	an excess of potassium in the blood
Hyperlipidemia	a general term meaning an excess of any or all kinds of lipids in the plasma
Hypernatremia	an excess of sodium in the blood
Hypochromic	a decrease of iron pigment in the red blood cells
Hypoglycemia	a condition in which the blood sugar level is too low
Hypokalemia	a decrease of potassium in the blood
Hyponatremia	a decrease of sodium in the blood
Hysterectomy	surgical removal of the uterus
Ileitis	inflammation of the ileum, which is the terminal portion of the small intestine
Immune	a condition in which the body is able to resist certain illnesses or toxins
Incubation	maintenance at a specified temperature and for a specified time period until growth or a reaction occurs

Word/Term	Meaning
Infarct	death of a segment of tissue, which results from a lack of blood supply to that area
Infection	invasion of the body by bacteria, molds, viruses, or parasites
Inoculate	to put into the body a substance (vaccine) that will cause the body to produce antibodies
Insulin	a natural hormone that is produced by the pancreas and is involved with the metabolism of blood sugar; diabetic individuals are not able to secrete proper amounts of their own insulin
Intercellular	located between the cells
Interstitial	pertains to that which occupies the space between the tissues
Ischemia	a temporary deficiency of blood to a localized area, which is caused by an obstruction
Isolation	the limitation of movement and social contact of a patient
Ketosis	an accumulation in the body of substances known as ketones, which may be detected by testing urine; it is commonly observed in patients who are starving or pregnant or have diabetes
Laryngitis	inflammation of the larynx
Leukemia	a blood disease in which there is an overproduction of white blood cells
Leukocytes	a broad term covering all types of white blood cells
Leukocytosis	an increase in the number of white blood cells
Leukopenia	a decrease in the number of white blood cells
Lipemic	the presence of an abnormal amount of fatty substance
Liter	a metric fluid measure of 1000 milliliters; approximately 2 pints

Word/Term	Meaning
Lithium	a psychoactive agent used in the treatment of manic-depressive disorders
Lysis	the dissolution of a red blood cell
Mastitis	inflammation of the breast
Megalocardia	enlarged heart
Melanoma	a malignant tumor that is often black
Menorrhagia	excessive menstrual flow
Metacarpal	having to do with the hands
Metatarsal	having to do with the feet
Microbiology	the study of microscopic organisms
Milliliter	1/1000 of a liter
Monilia	an outdated term indicating an infection with the yeast *Candida albicans;* candidiasis is the proper term
Morphology	the study of structure
Multiple myeloma	a disease characterized by the formation of multiple tumor masses in the bone and bone marrow
Multiple sclerosis	a chronic, slowly progressive disease of the nervous system
Myocarditis	inflammation of the heart muscle
Myxedema	a condition caused by the underfunctioning of the thyroid gland
Neonatal	the first 6 weeks after birth
Neoplasm	new growth (e.g., tumor)
Nephritis	inflammation of the kidney
Nephrology	science of the function and structure of the kidneys
Neurology	branch of medicine that deals with the nervous system and its diseases
Nosocomial	pertaining to a hospital; a nosocomial infection would be one obtained while in a hospital

Word/Term	Meaning
Obstetrics	branch of medicine concerned with women during pregnancy and childbirth
Oncology	branch of medicine that deals with tumors
Ophthalmology	branch of medicine that deals with the eye and its diseases
Orthopedic	branch of medicine that deals with problems of the skeleton, joints, muscles, and other supporting structures
Otitis	inflammation of the ear; the area is differentiated (e.g., otitis media means inflammation of the middle ear)
Otorrhea	a discharge from the ear
Palpate	to examine by touching with the fingers
Palpitation	a rapid intense beating of the heart
Pancreatitis	inflammation of the pancreas
Patent	open where fluid such as blood can flow freely; we say that a vein is patent if the vein still has its elasticity or if there is no blockage because of scar tissue
Pathogenic	anything that can produce a disease
Pathology	study of structural or functional changes in body tissues and organs caused by a disease
Pediatrics	branch of medicine related to the care and treatment of diseases of children
Pharyngitis	inflammation of the pharynx
Phlebitis	inflammation of a vein, which is often accompanied by clot formation
Prandial	pertains to a meal and is used in relation to timing, as in "2-hour postprandial" or 2 hours after a meal
Precision	to repeat a procedure several times and be able to obtain nearly the same answer every time

Word/Term	Meaning
Proctology	branch of medicine that deals with the diagnosis and treatment of diseases of the anus, rectum, and colon
Psychiatry	branch of medicine that deals with mental illness
Pulmonary	refers to the lungs and lung tissue
Renal	relating to the kidney
Respiratory	having to do with respiration or, more specifically, the taking in of oxygen and the release of carbon dioxide by the lungs
Rod	a nonspecific name for a group of bacteria that generally have the shape of a slender straight bar
Salpingitis	inflammation of the fallopian tubes
Sclerosis	a general term indicating the abnormal hardening of tissue
Sepsis	an infection of the blood with a pathogenic organism or a product (toxin) produced by the organism
Serology	the testing of blood serum for antigen-antibody reactions
Shunt	to divert flow from one main route to another
Sterile	the absence of living microorganisms
Susceptible	a condition in which a person is more than normally vulnerable to a disease
Syncope	a fainting spell
Thrombophlebitis	inflammation of the wall of a vein with an accompanying clot at the site
Thrombosis	the formation of a blood clot called a thrombus, which remains at the site of its formation in the circulatory system; when it becomes detached, it is known as an embolus
Transmission	the spreading of a disease from one person to another

Word/Term	*Meaning*
Transudate	a fluid that has diffused through the capillaries; it differs from an exudate in that it has fewer cellular elements
Urinary	having to do with the urinary tract or urine
Urology	branch of medicine concerned with the urinary tract of both sexes and the genital tract of males
Vaginitis	inflammation of the vagina
Vascular	refers to the blood system; also describes tissue heavily supplied with blood vessels
Vasoconstrictor	an agent that causes a decrease in the diameter of a blood vessel; this condition may be caused by either the introduction of a drug or a disease condition
Vasodilator	refers to an agent that causes an increase in the diameter of a blood vessel, thus producing greater blood flow
Virology	study of viruses, which are infectious agents that are too small to be seen through the usual light microscope

GENERAL ABBREVIATIONS

Abbreviations	*Meaning*
ac	before meals (*ante cibum*)
ad lib	as desired (*ad libitum*)
AIDS	acquired immunodeficiency syndrome
ASAP	as soon as possible
b.i.d.	twice a day (*bis in die*)
B/P	blood pressure
CA/Ca	cancer
cc	cubic centimeters
CLIA	Clinical Laboratories Improvement Act
CLS	Clinical Laboratory Scientist
CLT	Clinical Laboratory Technician
cm	centimeter

Abbreviations	*Meaning*
COPD	chronic obstructive pulmonary disease
CPR	cardiopulmonary resuscitation
CPT	Certified Phlebotomy Technician
CVA	cardiovascular or cerebrovascular accident
D & C	dilation and curettage
DO	Doctor of Osteopathy
DOA	dead on arrival
DOB	date of birth
ECG	electrocardiogram
EEG	electroencephalogram
EKG	electrocardiogram (ECG is the preferred abbreviation)
ENT	ear, nose, and throat
ER	emergency room
FUO	fever of unknown origin
GI	gastrointestinal
HCFA	Health Care Financing Administration
hs	hour of sleep
ICU	intensive care unit
IM	intramuscular (injection site)
I & O	intake and output
IV	intravenous
L	liter
LP	lumbar puncture
LPN	Licensed Practical Nurse
MD	Doctor of Medicine
MI	myocardial infarction
MLT	Medical Laboratory Technician
MRSA	methicillin-resistant *Staphylococcus aureus*
MS	multiple sclerosis
MSDS	material safety data sheets
MT	Medical Technologist
NPO	nothing by mouth (*non per os*)
OB	obstetrics
OD	overdose or overdosage
OR	operating room
OSHA	Occupational Safety and Health Administration
pc	after a meal (*post cibum*)
PDR	Physician's Desk Reference
Ph.D	Doctor of Philosophy
PP	postprandial (after a meal)
prn	as required (*pro re nata*)

Abbreviations	*Meaning*
qd	every day (*quaque die*)
qh	every hour (*quaque hora*)
q2h	every 2 hours (*quaque secunda hora*)
qid	four times daily (*quater in die*)
QNS	quantity not sufficient
qod	every other day (*quaque altera die*)
qs	as much as may suffice (*quantum sufficiat*)
RN	Registered Nurse
SBE	subacute bacterial endocarditis
SOB	shortness of breath
stat	to be done immediately (*statim*)
tid	three times a day (*ter in die*)
TPR	temperature/pulse/respiration
TUR	transurethral resection
URI	upper respiratory infection or illness
UTI	urinary tract infection
VRE	vancomycin-resistant enterococci

OFTEN USED CLINICAL LABORATORY ABBREVIATIONS

Abbreviations	*Meaning*
Ab	antibody
ABO	blood types
AFB	acid–fast bacillus
AFP	α-fetoprotein
ALT	alanine aminotransferase (SGPT)
ANA	antinuclear antibody
anti-HBc	hepatitis B core antibody
anti-HBe	hepatitis B e antibody
anti-HBs	hepatitis B surface antibody
APTT	activated partial thromboplastin time (PTT)
ASO	antistreptolysin-O
AST	aspartate aminotransferase (SGOT)
BT	bleeding time
BUN	blood urea nitrogen
C3/C4	complement
C50/C100	total complement
Ca	calcium

Abbreviations	Meaning
CBC	complete blood (cell) count
CEA	carcinoembryonic antigen
CMV	cytomegalovirus
CPK/CK	creatinine phosphokinase
CRP	C-reactive protein
CSF	cerebrospinal fluid
DIC	disseminated intravascular coagulopathy or coagulation
diff	white blood cell differential
EBV	Epstein-Barr virus
ESR	erythrocyte sedimentation rate
FBS	fasting blood sugar
FDP	fibrin degradation product
FSH	follicle-stimulating hormone
FTA	fluorescent treponemal antibody
GC	gonorrhea
g/dl	grams per deciliter
GTT	glucose tolerance test
HAA	hepatitis-associated antigen (HBsAg)
HAV	hepatitis A virus
HB_cAb	hepatitis B core antibody (anti-HBc)
HB_eAb	hepatitis B e antibody (anti-HBe)
HB_eAg	hepatitis B e antigen
HB_sAb	hepatitis B surface antibody (anti-HBs)
HB_sAg	hepatitis B surface antigen (HAA)
hCG	human chorionic gonadotropin
HCl	hydrochloric acid
Hct	hematocrit
HCV	hepatitis C virus (non-A, non-B hepatitis)
HDL	high-density lipoprotein (cholesterol)
HDV	hepatitis D (delta) virus
Hgb	hemoglobin
HIV	human immunodeficiency virus (the AIDS virus)
HLA	human leukocyte antigen
HPF	high-power field (microscopes)
HPL	human placental lactogen
HSV	herpes simplex virus
IU	International Unit
K	potassium
kg	kilogram
KOH	potassium hydroxide
LD/LDH	lactate dehydrogenase

Abbreviations	*Meaning*
LDL	low-density lipoprotein (cholesterol)
LE	lupus erythematosus
Li	lithium
LPF	low-power field (microscope)
MCH	mean corpuscular hemoglobin
MCHC	mean cell hemoglobin concentration
MCV	mean corpuscular volume
mEq/L	milliequivalent per liter
mg	milligram
ml/mL	milliliter
mm	millimeter
mm^3	cubic millimeter
Na	sodium
NaOH	sodium hydroxide
O&P	ova and parasites (stool examination)
PAP	prostatic acid phosphatase
Pap	Papanicolaou stain
PKU	phenylketonuria
PSA	prostate-specific antigen
PT	prothrombin time
PTT	partial thromboplastin time (APTT)
RBC	red blood (cell) count
retic	reticulocyte
Rh	blood factor (Rhesus) reported as negative or positive, usually with the blood type (e.g., O positive)
RMSF	Rocky Mountain spotted fever
RPR	rapid plasma reagent (test for syphilis)
RSV	respiratory syncytial virus
sed rate	sedimentation rate
SGOT	serum glutamic-oxaloacetic transaminase (AST)
SGPT	serum glutamic-pyruvic transaminase (ALT)
SLE	systemic lupus erythematosus
SMA	sequential multichannel autoanalyzer; smooth muscle antibody or autoantibody
STD	sexually transmitted disease
STS	serologic test (for) syphilis
TB	tuberculosis
TIBC	total iron-binding capacity
TP	total protein
TSH	thyroid-stimulating hormone
UA	urinalysis; uric acid

Abbreviations	*Meaning*
VDRL	Veneral Disease Research Laboratory (test for syphilis)
VLDL	very-low-density lipoprotein (cholesterol)
WBC	white blood (cell) count
X-match	cross match of blood for transfusion

SYMBOLS

Symbol	*Meaning*
$\bar{c}$	with
Pco_2	blood gas symbol—partial pressure of carbon dioxide
Po_2	blood gas symbol—partial pressure of oxygen
$\bar{s}$	without
μ	micron
↑	elevated
↓	decreased
>	greater than
<	less than
≥	equal to or greater than
≤	equal to or less than
≅	approximately equal to
D_x	diagnosis
R_x	prescription
1+	slight trace
2+	trace
3+	moderate
4+	large amount
$\mathbf{D}_x$	diagnosis

COMMONLY ORDERED LABORATORY TESTS

Test	*Basic Clinical Usefulness*
Acid phosphatase	detects prostatic cancer
Alanine aminotransferase (ALT/SGPT)	detects hepatic disease
Alkaline phosphatase	detects skeletal disease and hepatic disorders

Test	Basic Clinical Usefulness
α-fetoprotein (AFP)	assists in diagnosis of hepatic disorders and some neural tube congenital defects
Ammonia	detects severe hepatic disease
Amylase	detects pancreatitis
Antinuclear antibody (ANA)	screens for autoimmune disease, SLE, and chronic active hepatitis
Antistreptolysin O titer (ASO)	documents exposure to streptococcal infection
Aspartate amino-transferase (AST/SGOT)	detects acute hepatic disease and recent myocardial infarction
Bilirubin	evaluates liver function and aids in diagnosis of hemolytic anemia and biliary obstruction
Bleeding time	assesses hemostatic function
Blood culture	diagnoses bacteremia
Blood urea nitrogen (BUN)	evaluates renal function
Calcium	detects neuromuscular, skeletal, and endocrine disorders; blood-clotting deficiencies; and acid-base imbalance
Cardiac isoenzymes	rules out coronary heart disease
Cholesterol	assesses risk of coronary heart disease
Complete blood count (CBC)(includes red and white blood count)	assesses hemoglobin and hematocrit levels and provides differential diagnosis
Coombs'	the direct Coombs' detects proteins (antibodies) that coat the red blood cell; the indirect Coombs' detects for antibodies in serum
C-reactive protein	detects inflammation
Creatinine	assesses glomerular filtration
Creatinine phospho-kinase (CK/CPK)	diagnoses acute myocardial infarction

Test	*Basic Clinical Usefulness*
Electrolytes (sodium, potassium, chloride, carbon dioxide)	detects acid-base balance
Ferritin	assists in diagnosis of certain anemias and evaluates total body storage of iron
Fibrin degradation products (FDP)	helps in diagnosing DIC
Folic acid	evaluates certain anemias and detects deficiency because folic acid is important in metabolic energy-related processes
γ-glutamyltransferase (GGT)	helps in diagnosing obstructive jaundice, carcinoma of pancreas and liver, and chronic alcoholic liver disease
Glucose (fasting blood sugar) (FBS)	screens for diabetes mellitus
Glucose tolerance test (GTT)	confirms diabetes mellitus or hypoglycemia
Hematocrit	helps in diagnosing anemia
Hemoglobin	measures severity of anemia
Human chorionic gonadotropin (hCG)	tests for pregnancy
Iron	provides differential diagnosis of certain anemias
Lactic dehydrogenase (LD/LDH)	provides differential diagnosis of myocardial or pulmonary infarction, anemia, and hepatic disease
Lipase	diagnoses pancreatitis
Lipid profile	evaluates hyperlipidemia
Osmolality, serum	evaluates electrolyte levels, water balance, hydration states, and liver disease
Partial thromboplastin time (PTT/APTT)	screens for clotting factor deficiencies

Test	Basic Clinical Usefulness
Phenylketonuria (PKU)	screens for PKU levels in newborns for the prevention of mental retardation
Phosphorus	evaluates alcoholism and detects parathyroid and kidney disease
Platelet count	evaluates platelet production
Prostate-specific antigen (PSA)	levels correlate with extent of prostate cancer
Protein	detects hepatic disease, protein deficiency, and renal disorders
Prothrombin time (PT)	evaluates extrinsic coagulation
Rapid plasma reagent (RPR)	assists in diagnosis of syphilis
Red blood count (RBC)	supports other tests in diagnosis of anemia
Reticulocyte count	evaluates red blood cell production
Sickle cell preparation	detects sickle cell disease
T_3/T_4	evaluates thyroid function
Thyroid-stimulating hormone (TSH)	evaluates thyroid function
Total iron-binding capacity (TIBC)	provides differential diagnosis of certain anemias
Triglycerides	detects hyperlipidemia
Uric acid	detects gout and kidney dysfunction
White cell count (WBC)	detects inflammation or infection

BIBLIOGRAPHY

Burtis CA, Ashwood ER, eds. Tietz textbook of clinical chemistry, 2nd ed. Philadelphia: WB Saunders, 1994.

Dacunha JP, Ford RD, Glover SM, eds. Diagnostic. Springfield, IL: Intermed Communications, 1981.

Garb S. Laboratory tests in common use, 6th ed. New York: Springer, 1976.

Hamilton HD, ed. Definitions. Springhouse, PA: Intermed Communications, 1983.

Handbook of current medical abbreviations. Bowie, MD: The Charles Press, 1976.

Jacobs DS, Kasten BL Jr, DeMott WR, et al, eds. Laboratory test handbook, 2nd ed. Baltimore: Williams & Wilkins, 1990.

Kaplan LA, Pesce AJ. Clinical chemistry: theory, analysis, and correlation, 3rd ed. St. Louis, MO: Mosby, 1996.

McClatchey KD, ed. Clinical laboratory medicine. Baltimore: Williams & Wilkins, 1994

Smith GL, Davis PE. Medical terminology, 4th ed. New York: John Wiley and Sons, 1981.

Stedman's medical dictionary, 25th ed. Baltimore: Williams & Wilkins, 1990.

Stegeman W. Medical terms simplified. St. Paul, MN: West Publications, 1976.

Health Care Settings

Today, many different types of health care are offered in an ever-growing list of environments. Because all people need health care at some point, many different types of locations now offer health care that focuses on filling a specific health care need. Although there is much variation in how health care is specifically delivered in each, we will discuss only the basic organization found in each health care setting.

HOSPITALS

Hospitals serve as the foundation for health care. The primary focus of health care delivered in hospitals is oriented toward recovery of the sick patient. In hospitals, the sick and injured receive various treatments designed to restore health. Hospitals organize themselves into departments that optimize the various types of treatments physicians may need to order for patient recovery. The departments that are described below form the basic organization found within a hospital.

Nursing

Nursing is the health care service most commonly associated with hospitals. This profession offers education and training that is designed to provide the skills required to adequately care for sick people. Nursing education and training can range from courses taught in technical colleges to various levels of degrees (Bachelor of Science in Nursing [BSN], Master of Science in Nursing [MSN], Doctor of Philosophy [PhD], Doctor of Nursing [ND]). Some nursing positions require intense and specialized training. Examples of the specialized training that are available in nursing are operating room (OR), midwifery, and dialysis nurses. Other positions such as the floor nurse position require broader and general nursing knowledge. Patient Service Technicians and Patient Care Technicians provide basic nursing services for patients such as help with personal care. Some nursing positions are educational or administrative. Infectious disease nurses use their nursing knowledge to help control the spread of nosocomial infections. A Director of Nurses controls how the techniques of nursing are used in a health care facility. Education nurses provide appropriate continuing education classes to the nursing staff.

A Registered Nurse (RN) usually administers the vast array of procedures involved in direct patient care nursing. Licensed Practical Nurse (LPN) certification indicates an intermediate level of training. Patient Service and Patient Care Technicians complete their tasks under the guidance of an RN or LPN.

Laboratory

Hospital laboratories are regarded as an allied health care department within a hospital. This reinforces the basic idea of ancillary hospital departments that join together for the benefit of the patient. Other allied health care departments may include those departments, such as Radiology, Physical Therapy, and Speech Therapy, whose treatments call for them to come in direct contact with patients. A laboratory provides important diagnostic information to physicians on specimens that are collected from patients.

Laboratory specimens can range from those that are commonly collected (e.g., blood and urine) to those that require direct sampling by physicians (e.g., tissue samples). Laboratory instruments are used to precisely measure patient samples for various analytes. Laboratory instrumentation used to test patient samples is closely monitored for accuracy by using quality control (QC). Here, known samples are tested for accuracy to ensure proper test results on unknown patient samples. Laboratory test results are made available to physicians and other health care workers who are directly involved with patient care in a variety of ways. Results can be posted in the traditional way of charting results on a patient's chart or through a computer where the results can either be viewed on a screen or printed out on demand.

The staff in a laboratory can be trained at many levels. Training is available at the baccalaureate level (Medical Technologist or Clinical Laboratory Scientist) or the associate degree level (Medical Laboratory Technician or Clinical Laboratory Technician). Increasingly, more **phlebotomists and laboratory sup**port technicians are receiving limited technical training and on-the-job instruction that is tied to their laboratory duties. Some Medical Technologists are certified at the specialist level in a single department of laboratory work, such as Hematology, Chemistry, Blood Bank, or Microbiology. Other Medical Technologists who retain a basic knowledge in all areas are known as Generalists. Advanced degrees such as Master's degrees (MAs) and PhDs are available in some specialized areas of Medical Technology including clinical microbiology, immunology, and clinical chemistry. A physician who specializes in laboratory work is a Pathologist. The areas of specialization in the areas of pathology are anatomic pathology, forensic pathology, and cytopathology. Workers who scan slides for cellular abnormalities under the direction of a pathologist are cytologists. Those who assist pathologists by cutting and staining tissue samples are histologists.

X-Ray

Another allied health department providing diagnostic information is X-Ray. Here, images or pictures are taken of a patient's body using ionizing radiation or x-rays. These pictures allow physicians to view the shape of internal structures. The evolution of other imaging techniques in addition to x-rays has caused this department to often be renamed Radiology or Medical Imaging. Here, other patient imaging techniques that use sound waves, computers, or magnetic fields allow the internal organs in a body to be highlighted or outlined on film.

Workers in this field who have received 2 years of technical training in Radiology are registered as Radiologic Technologists. Radiology Technologists who undergo additional non-technical training at the baccalaureate level obtain a BSRT degree. The X-Ray staff with only on-the-job training must undergo a continuing education course required by many states to ensure the safe use of radiation. A physician who specializes in reading and interpreting radiology film and other imaging techniques that are used in special situations is called a Radiologist.

Pharmacy

After diagnosing a disease, physicians may treat a patient's condition by administering medications. The pharmacy is responsible for preparing any medications that are given to patients in a hospital. Here, pharmacists gauge the appropriateness of medications ordered, prepare medications by weighing and mixing ingredients, and deliver proper dosing to the nursing floors responsible for administering the medications to patients. Pharmacists have college degrees and training that teaches them to prepare and dispense medications safely. Pharmacy technicians receive training at the associate degree level, which allows them to dispense all drugs under the direct guidance of a pharmacist. Many pharmacy technicians have a background in health care that provides some familiarity with medications.

Physical, Occupational, Respiratory, and Speech Therapy

Some health care is rehabilitative in nature and serves to restore the health of people who are recuperating from debilitating illnesses. These services allow people to recuperate outside the traditional hospital setting and have access to health care and monitoring that is not available in the home. Rehabilitation departments offer specific types of treatment tailored to the specialized needs of patients. Physical Therapists are college graduates with education and training in preparing and guiding patients whose mobility has been limited. They have knowledge of muscle function and movement and bone and joint structure. A degree in Occupational Therapy allows Occupational Therapists to help patients achieve a normal lifestyle after a debilitating illness or injury. Respiratory Therapists work with patients whose ability to breathe normally has been altered. Often respiratory therapists provide diagnostic information to physicians by collecting and performing a blood gas test. Respiratory Therapists are trained with a college degree and have a complete understanding of respiration. Respiratory Technicians receive technical training at the associate degree level. Speech Therapists have training beyond the baccalaureate level and help patients regain the ability to speak normally after illness or injury. A Speech Therapist knows the anatomy of the mouth, neck, and jaw and helps patients with the mouth and jaw movements necessary for swallowing.

Medical Records

Imagine keeping track of all the information produced as medical care is delivered to hospitalized patients. The department responsible for maintaining this extensive data is Medical Records. Other names hospitals have given to this department include Information Management Department and Health Information Services.

Regardless of the name, this department is responsible for storing and maintaining the massive amount of documentation generated during hospitalization. New computer technology aids this department in such tasks as records analysis and transcription. Other tasks include coding for correct reimbursement from the government, maintaining awareness of new laws and regulations concerning information management, and joining other health care departments in striving to improve service to customers by using quality improvement plans.

Various types of education are needed to fill positions in Medical Records. Transcriptionists and staff performing chart assembly require no special training. Technical workers receive an Associate Degree in Records Technology. Management positions are held by those with a baccalaureate degree in Registered Records Administration. A Certified Coding Specialist degree can be obtained by receiving further auxiliary training in this field. To maintain the confidentiality of medical records, usually any person releasing medical information has a notary public license.

Dietary

Hospitals must be careful about the food and beverages patients receive while hospitalized. The digestive systems of hospitalized patients may not be able to process certain food items without harm. Registered Dietitians are certified with formal training in nutrition and decide the menus of hospital food based upon the dietary requirements of patients. Physicians may refer their patients to a Nutritionist who guides patients in appropriate diets for the maintenance of health after release from their hospital stay.

PUBLIC HEALTH

Some health care is designed to be preventative in nature. This type of health care is extended as a service to the public and serves to maintain the public's general health. Examples of this type of service include mass health screenings for increased blood sugar levels and elevated blood pressure. This type of health care screens for health problems that are just beginning or that are otherwise undetected.

Health care offered to the general public is also made available by state and federally funded health agencies who offer the public basic health services and sanitation control, personal hygiene education, and infectious disease control. These agencies also provide general health education to the public at large. An example of this type of education includes the programs designed to educate young mothers in the importance of prenatal health care.

BLOOD DONATION

An important area of health care that is often overlooked is blood or blood product donation. Blood donors are screened for their suitability to donate by answering questions about their health, lifestyle, and personal habits. After being found suitable, potential donors have their vital signs checked. This multilevel process of screening helps ensure a safe blood supply for the injured or sick patient who needs a blood transfusion for recovery. After donation, the blood or blood product is tested for various diseases that can be transmitted by transfusion.

The screening process for the donation process of pheresis is slightly more stringent than the requirement for whole blood donation. In this process, whole blood is continuously drawn from a donor's arm and proceeds into a pheresis machine through intravenous (IV) tubing. The pheresis instrument continuously centrifuges the blood, which causes red blood cells to separate from the plasma they are floating in as well as the donor's white blood cells. After this separation occurs, the plasma or white blood cells are partially removed and collected in a sterile bag. The donor's remaining blood is then returned on a continual basis from the pheresis machine to the donor through the IV tubing. This continual cycle ensures that pheresis donors actually experience little blood loss. For this reason, donors may undergo the pheresis process more frequently then they are able to donate whole blood.

HOME HEALTH CARE

Patients with a variety of medical conditions that may have caused previous hospitalization are now cared for successfully in their homes. Some patients that are released from hospitals need some form of managed care at home to complete their recovery. Home health organizations offer a variety of services for the home-bound patient and provide health education that may be needed by the patient for complete recovery. Home health care is ordered by a patient's physician when the patient is released from the hospital. For those with an ongoing medical condition, this means continued hospitalization can be avoided by receiving treatments from health care workers in the home on a continual basis. Home health care has become a fast growing segment of the health care market. Because of the rising cost of medical care, many HMOs and insurance companies are choosing to finance basic health care that can be provided for patients in their homes.

NURSING HOMES

Because of a rise in population coupled with increased life expectancy, nursing homes now house an increasing number of older Americans who are unable to receive adequate care at home. Also, recent advances in medical science and medical technology have resulted in the saving of lives of seriously ill patients who partially recover but need care that is unavailable to them in the home. These situations have resulted in an increased demand for the type of health care provided by nursing homes where workers who are trained in health care provide the skills necessary for assistance with the elderly or those unable to care for themselves. Nursing home populations vary from those needing little assistance to those who are completely dependent. Health care work in these facilities therefore ranges from basic patient care and phlebotomy to various nursing skills ordered by the patient's physician that are provided by LPNs and RNs and coordinated by a senior nurse.

PHYSICIANS' OFFICES

A physician's office provides health care that is specifically oriented toward assisting patients who visit the doctor because of a health care complaint. The manner and technical complexity of this assistance depend upon the type of medicine a physician specializes in and how many special procedures are required. Some physicians who offer only specialized care may only require competent clerical help and basic patient care technicians, while those physicians offering basic care need to perform a wider range of treatments for a multitude of health problems. The staff in a physician's office may vary from on-the-job trained Patient Care Technicians to Nurse Practitioners (NP) and Physicians Assistants (PA).

DIALYSIS

Dialysis treatment centers are used to treat patients who are experiencing kidney failure. This means that the patient's kidneys are, because of a variety of disease states, unable to cleanse the patient's blood of waste materials. The waste materials that are present in blood are not the solid waste we might imagine but are chemical constituents in the blood that are the waste products of the cellular metabolism. Normally, the kidneys filter blood to remove these products that are excreted in urine. If this chemical waste builds up to intolerable levels in the bloodstream, the patient slips into a coma and dies.

For dialysis, blood is withdrawn from veins via IV tubing into a dialysis machine where the blood is filtered and cleansed before being returned to the patient. Since this process occurs continuously, a patient's entire volume of blood can be cleansed in a matter of hours. Patients need to receive dialysis at least twice weekly or the waste levels build up to dangerous levels. For this reason, patients who undergo dialysis on a routine basis have shunts placed in their arms, which protect and allow easier access to the veins that are used in this life-saving procedure. Patients receiving dialysis usually are cared for by a RN who has received special training in the dialysis procedure.

VETERINARY TECHNICIANS

Historically, specific education or training for veterinary technicians has not been required; however, times have changed. Today veterinary technology is a profession with specific skills. Oftentimes, a veterinary technician functions as a nurse, a medical technologist, a radiology technician, a dental hygienist, a pharmacist, an anesthetist, an electrocardiogram (ECG) technician, a surgery technician, a computer operator, and an inventory specialist. Veterinary technicians take animal x-rays, give injections, read blood tests, assist in veterinary surgery, clean teeth, anesthetize animal patients, and give postoperative care. These workers form the backbone of a veterinary clinic staff allowing the doctor to concentrate on medical issues of animal patients. At least 36 states now license veterinary technicians with schooling that requires at least 2 years of education and training.

BIBLIOGRAPHY

Alberson K. Training medical records personnel. Personal Interview. November 13, 1997; Tifton, GA.

Amended, BSD 51.110, Blood donor interview, processing, and management. Washington, DC: American Red Cross, 1996.

Dampier Connie, RN. Aspects of home health nursing. Personal interview: August 13, 1997; Tifton, GA.

Ellis A. Training of radiology workers. Personal interview: August 29, 1997; Tifton, GA.

Department of Physical Therapy, College of Wisconsin: Department of Philosophy. Available at http://jeffline.tju.edu/CWIS/DEPT/PT/npt.html. Accessed September 1, 1997.

Dog Owners Guide, Veterinary Technicians. Available at http://www.canismajpr.com/dog/vettech.html. Accessed August 13, 1997.

Opus Communications Healthwave—Medical Records Briefing. Available at http://www.opuscomm.com/nls/indeces/mrbx.html. Accessed November 13, 1997.

University of Washington Curriculum in Physical Therapy (PT), UW Rehabilitation Medicine. Available at http:\\weber.u.washongtpm.edu/~rehab/pt/bs.html. Accessed September 1, 1997.

Weathersby H, RPH, Pharm D. Pharmacy education. Personal interview. September 4, 1997; Nashville, GA.

Legal and Regulatory Issues

LEGAL ISSUES

For most health care professionals and health care institutions, a great deal of energy has been concentrated on the delivery of health care using the latest concepts and technologies. But new laws and ethical questions have come with these rapidly changing concepts and technologies. This has resulted in a multitude of challenges to the way health care is administered and inevitable litigations or lawsuits. Although it is hoped that those reading this text will never have the experience of a lawsuit, nevertheless, it is prudent for health care professionals to be aware of what occurs and also be knowledgeable of some basic actions that can be done to help avoid the unpleasantness of a litigation. Following is a discussion generally describing what to expect if a lawsuit occurs. The example assumes that any alleged harm was not willfully done. *Remember, lawsuits are always to be taken seriously.*

Legal Terms It Is Helpful To Know

Affidavit: A statement or testimony

Ante litem: Before litigation; a notice that must be sent to a government institution or employee, which gives the institution or employee an opportunity to "do the right thing" before a lawsuit is filed

Appeal: Request that a case be heard by a higher court in order to seek review and hopefully reversal of a lower court's ruling

Arbiter: A person, such as a judge, who is empowered to decide matters that are at issue

Battery: Touching a person against their will or without their consent

Breach of duty: Duty means responsibility or obligation to the patient. It is a breach of duty if whatever harm was done to the patient could have been avoided.

Compensation/Compensatory damages: Compensatory damages are meant to compensate the plaintiff for some harm suffered because of an action or inaction by the defendant.

Defendant: The party accused by the plaintiff of having harmed him or her in some manner

Demand-letter: A letter that may be sent before a lawsuit is filed stating that the party receiving the letter is liabel for some act and requesting compensation

Deposition: This is a type of pre-trial discovery in which attorneys for both the defendant and plaintiff will, in question-and-answer form, take the statement of a witness.

Discovery: Discovery is a time period in a lawsuit where the lawyers for both the plaintiff and defendant gather information in preparation for a possible trial. Two principle means of discovery are depositions and interrogatories.

Interrogatory: Like the deposition, this is a type of pre-trial discovery in which written questions are sent to a witness who makes a reply under oath. Unlike the deposition, there is not an opportunity for cross-examination.

Liable: Being responsible for damages

Litigation: Lawsuit

Malpractice: When care is given to a patient in an unprofessional or unskillful way

Negligence: When care given to a patient is not given according to acceptable standards of practice

Plaintiff: The party that is initiating a lawsuit

Summary judgment: A judgment without the necessity of a jury trial

Ultra vires: Beyond legal authority

An Overview of What to Expect if a Lawsuit Occurs

The first thing that could happen is that the health care professional or institution would get a **demand-letter.** More than likely it would be a registered letter with a return receipt requested. It might say something like this:

Dear Health Care Professional or Health Care Institution:
We believe you have damaged our client Mr. Jones. On January 1 of this year you attempted a venipuncture, which went through the vein. Because of this, our client suffers from complete numbness of the left arm and continual migraine headaches. We believe you are liable for this. Our client is 42 years old and was an engineer at the National Aeronautics and Space Administration. He made an annual salary of $200,000. Because of the events mentioned above, he can no longer be gainfully employed, he has incurred numerous medical expenses, not to mention the mental

anguish and suffering by his family. Since we believe you to be liable, we think he
should be compensated for the amount of 10 million dollars.
Signed:
Mr. Jones' Lawyer

Circumstances vary, but in most cases the party receiving the **demand-letter** would not respond. If our Mr. Jones still felt that there has been a harmful act against him and he should be compensated, then a lawsuit would be filed.

If a lawsuit is filed, it will be delivered to the defendant personally by either a deputy sheriff or a process-server. Often included with the lawsuit is an affidavit by some expert in the field who states that the action taken by the health care professional or institution was somehow out of the norm, inappropriate, or was not done according to accepted standards of practice. Unlike the demand-letter, *the lawsuit must not be ignored!* If the defendant chooses not to answer the lawsuit, the defendant will lose by default whether guilty or not. One intervening item: if the health care professional or institution is a governmental agency, they might enjoy a degree of sovereign immunity. Before a lawsuit is filed an **anti litem** notice would be sent. This must be done before a lawsuit can be filed against a governmental agency.

After the lawsuit is filed, the **discovery** phase begins. This could include **depositions** and **interrogatories.** In addition, there may be a **subpoena** for either records or procedure and policy manuals. In some cases, after the discovery phase has been completed, one of the parties involved in the lawsuit may make a motion for a **summary judgment.** This is a motion made by either the plaintiff's or defendant's lawyer setting out all the reasons to win without a trial. Essentially, the motion states that both sides agree that there are no differences in the facts and the facts are such that either the plaintiff or the defendant should prevail. In a summary judgment the judge is the sole **arbiter.** The decision of the judge, however, can be **appealed.**

If the lawsuit for various reasons is not settled out of court but goes to trial, it must be realized that both sides are "playing the cards." The plaintiff and the defendant have already been asked everything that is relative to the case. The lawyers for both parties know what the cards are, they are simply presenting the data to a jury and letting the jury make the call.

Suggestions to Help Prevent Litigation

As implied earlier in this chapter, lawsuits are no fun. They can be time-consuming and worrisome. While there are no guarantees, the following are actions that can help prevent the possibility of a lawsuit.

1. Always be empathetic toward patients. If, for example, a hematoma forms while doing a venipuncture, show proper concern and explain to the pa-

tient what they can do to treat the hematoma. Follow-up may even be appropriate. Never, however, quickly admit fault. You may not be guilty of poor standard of practice. The hematoma may have formed no matter how excellent your technique.
2. Always respect and protect patients' confidentiality. Never discuss patient information where others can hear you. Remember that medical information, verbal or written, should be accessible only to those who "need to know" in order to give effective patient care.
3. Perform only those procedures that you are trained and approved to do.
4. Meticulously follow the most recent procedure and policy manuals of the health care institution where you are employed.
5. Maintain accurate, complete, and up-to-date records, logs, and quality assurance documentation.
6. Last but not least, as was stated in the chapter on professionalism, the health care professional who appears unhurried, who is considerate and gentle when handling the patient, and who speaks in an authoritative but quiet voice, further enhances the patient's confidence in that health care professional.

REGULATORY ISSUES

Approximately 12,000 hospitals and independent laboratories became regulated under the Clinical Laboratory Improvement Act passed by Congress in 1967. Then in 1988, after congressional hearings revealed serious deficiencies in the quality of physician office laboratories and in Pap smear testing, Congress passed the Clinical Laboratory Improvement Amendment (CLIA). This amendment unified and replaced previous standards with a single set of requirements that applied to all laboratories testing human specimens. The key feature of the new regulations was the new classification testing level according to method complexity. Four levels of testing complexity have been defined: Waived Testing, Practitioner Performed Microscopy, Moderate Complexity Testing, and High Complexity Testing. Briefly outlined below are the requirements for each of the categories. It should be pointed out that in addition to the CLIA '88 regulations, some states have laws that regulate clinical laboratories and the personnel that may perform clinical laboratory testing in that state.

Waived Testing

1. Must apply for a certificate of waiver (Health Care Finance Administration (HCFA) 116 Form)
2. No qualifications for testing personnel
3. Must follow manufacturer's instructions
4. No routine governmental agency inspections
5. Testing is limited to simple procedures for which the likelihood of error is negligible and which pose minimal harm if performed incorrectly.

Practitioner-Performed Microscopy

1. Must apply for a Practitioner-Performed Microscopy (PPM) certificate of waiver (HCFA 116 Form)
2. Tests must be performed by a physician, nurse practitioner, nurse mid-wife, or physician's assistant.
3. Must follow the moderate complexity requirements for quality control, quality assurance, proficiency testing (if available), and patient test management
4. No routine governmental agency inspections.
5. Testing is limited to:
   - All wet-mount preparations for the presence or absence of bacteria, fungi, parasites, and human cellular elements
   - KOH preparations
   - Fern tests
   - Pinworm examinations
   - Post-coital direct qualitative examinations of vaginal or cervical mucus
   - Urine sedimentation examinations
   - Nasal smear examinations for granulocytes
   - Fecal leukocyte examinations
   - Qualitative semen analysis (limited to the presence or absence of sperm and detection of motility)

Moderate Complexity Testing

1. Must register as a moderate complex testing laboratory (HCFA 116 Form)
2. Personnel must include a laboratory director, clinical consultant, technical consultant, and testing personnel. Minimum qualifications for testing personnel are a high school diploma or equivalent and documented training.
3. Special requirements:
   a) Must be enrolled in an approved proficiency testing program for each regulated analyte tested
   b) A procedure manual for all methods must be readily available.
   c) A quality control program that includes calibration at least every 6 months of instruments or systems that can be calibrated, run and document two levels of controls each day of patient testing, and document remedial actions taken as a result of errors or control results
   d) Patient test management documentation covering requisitions, records proving that an ordered test was performed, testing reporting, referral testing, and a protocol for collecting and processing specimens
   e) A quality assurance program that monitors and evaluates the quality of service provided
4. Routine inspections

5. Testing:
   - Most hematology instruments
   - Manual differential limited to the identification of normal cells only
   - Most chemistry tests
   - Urine culture for colony count only
   - Urethral and cervical Gram's stain for gonorrhea
   - Throat culture screen
   - Microscopic urinalysis
   - Rapid kits for streptococcus, mononucleosis, serum pregnancy, and Chlamydia

High Complexity Testing

1. Must register as a high complex testing laboratory (HCFA 116 Form)
2. Personnel include a laboratory director, clinical consultant, technical supervisor, general supervisor, and testing personnel. Minimum qualification for testing personnel is an associate degree in laboratory science or previously qualified technologist.
3. Special requirements are the same as for moderate complex testing with the addition of method and calibration verification.
4. Routine inspections
5. Testing includes everything in moderate complex testing and the following additions:
   - Manual hematology counts
   - Complete identification of abnormal cells in the manual differential
   - Non-automated chemistry
   - Gram's stains from any source
   - Microbiologic cultures from any source, organism identification, and antimicrobial susceptibility testing
   - Quantitative semen analysis

BIBLIOGRAPHY

American Research Corporation. Glossary of Legal Terms and Phrases. Available at http://www.lawlead.com/common/glossary.html. Accessed June 26, 1997.

Ellis R. What a health care worker may expect during a lawsuit. Personal interview: July 24, 1997; Nashville, GA.

Faber V. Understanding medicolegal issues. Key to avoid phlebotomy malpractice suits. Advance 7(5):10, 1995

Federal Register. 57(40):7218, February 28, 1992

Federal Register. 58(11):5212, January 19, 1993

Federal Register. 60(78):20035, April 24, 1995

Root C. Complying with CLIA '88. Westwood, MA: Behring Diagnostics, Inc., 1995.

St. Hill H. Legislation and Medico Legal Issues Affecting Phlebotomy Practice. ASCP Fall Teleconference Series, Oct. 17, 1995.

General Rules for Infection Prevention and Safety

INFECTION PREVENTION

Alone, no approach is 100% effective to protect against infection from blood-borne pathogens.

The use of personal protective equipment, employee work practices, and

adherence to safety standards, engineering controls, vaccination, and training must

all be used together.

Diseases that are transmitted from one person (or animal) to another person are called **communicable diseases** or **infections.** The transmission of the agent of an infectious disease from its source to a susceptible individual is called the **chain of infection.** This chain of infection (source of infection → a means of transmission → susceptible host) may be broken anywhere along its links by sterilization, immunization, aseptic techniques, handwashing, the wearing of gloves, and isolation procedures.

Infectious disease agents may be transmitted by several routes, and the same infectious agent may be transmitted by more than one route. In general, however, there are five main routes in which infectious microorganisms are transmitted.

1. **Droplet transmission** in which droplets containing microorganisms are propelled a short distance through the air and deposited on a susceptible individual's eyes, nasal mucosa, or mouth. Although coughing and sneezing most often come to mind when thinking of droplet transmissions, centrifugation and the "popping" of specimen container tops are also responsible for droplet formation.
2. **Airborne transmission** should not be confused with droplet transmission. Airborne transmission occurs by the dissemination of either micro-droplets or droplets that have evaporated and still contain microorganisms. Unlike

the droplets mentioned in item 1, these droplets remain suspended in the air for long periods of time. Thus, infectious agents carried in this manner can be dispersed by air currents and can be inhaled by a susceptible individual in close proximity (e.g., in the same room) and even over longer distances depending on environmental conditions. Examples of this type of transmission include Mycobacterium tuberculosis and some fungal infections.

3. **Contact transmission** can be **direct** or **indirect.** In **direct** contact, the causative agent is passed from one individual directly to another individual. In other words, a direct body-membrane-to-body-membrane contact. Infections with syphilis, gonorrhea, hepatitis B virus (HBV), and human immunodeficiency virus (HIV), which causes acquired immunodeficiency syndrome (AIDS), are commonly contracted in this manner. So too are staphylococcal infections because this bacterium can be transferred from the hands of one person to the skin surface of another during patient-care activities that require personal contact. Hand contact, such as "shaking hands" with an infected individual, is also thought to be a primary way that respiratory virus infections are spread. Individuals can be **indirectly** exposed to infectious agents through contact with **inanimate objects.** Examples of this include blood collection tubes, specimen containers, telephone handsets, and pencils and pens that are contaminated on the outside with infected blood or body substances. Accidental needle sticks and gloves that are not changed between patients are other examples. Also included in this type of transmission is the sharing of needles by drug abusers.

4. **Vehicle transmission** applies to microorganisms transmitted by contaminated items such as food, water, and medications. Salmonellosis and Shigellosis in food, hepatitis A and Salmonellosis in water, and hemolytic Escherichia coli in poorly cooked meat are examples of infectious agents spread in this manner.

5. **Vector-borne transmission** occurs when an arthropod, referred to as a vector, transfers an organism. Examples of vector-borne transmission are malaria and encephalitis, which are transmitted by mosquitoes, and Lyme disease and Rocky Mountain Spotted Fever, which are spread by ticks.

Infections that may be contracted outside of a health care setting are called **community-acquired infections.** Coming down with the flu is an example of this type of infection. **Nosocomial infections** are infections that may be acquired by an individual *after* admission into a health care setting. This type of infection is most often caused by improper precautions used by health care workers when going from one patient to another. New in the lexicon but similar in cause are **nosohusial infections.** These are infections that are acquired in the course of home care.

Body Substance Isolation, Universal Precautions, and OSHA Blood-Borne Pathogen Rules

Developed in the early 1980s, **Body Substance Isolation** (BSI) defined *all* body fluids and substances as infectious. BSI was designed to reduce cross-transmission of organisms among patients and to reduce the exposure of health care workers to moist body substances of patients. Its strategy was to focus on tasks and procedures and not the diagnosis of the patient.

In 1985, largely because of the HIV epidemic, the Centers for Disease Control (CDC) recommended a new aggressive standardized approach to infection control termed **"Universal Precautions"** (UP). This new strategy was mandated into standards by the Occupational Safety and Health Administration (OSHA) on December 6, 1991. The purpose of these standards was to protect all employees who might reasonably anticipate being occupationally-exposed to blood and other potentially infectious materials. According to the concept of UP, all human blood and certain body fluids are to be treated as if they contain HIV, HBV, or other blood borne pathogens. Under the OSHA guidelines, after a task has been categorized for possible exposure to blood borne pathogens, strategies for controlling hazards and reducing the risk of exposure must be developed. These strategies, which are discussed in the sections below, include work practice controls, personal protective equipment (PPE), housekeeping, training, administration of the hepatitis B vaccine, and engineering controls.

HANDWASHING

Of all the safety precautions available in a health care setting, handwashing is the easiest to perform, but unfortunately also seems to be the easiest for health care workers to ignore. Proper washing of the hands is the most effective tool against the spread of disease caused by microorganisms. Each year there are more than 2,400,000 nosocomial infections in the United States. It is estimated that these nosocomial infections directly cause 30,000 deaths with an average cost per incident of $2,300 and an overall cost of $4.5 billion annually in extended care and treatment. The CDC estimates that each year there are more than 1.5 million nosocomial infections in extended care facilities, and the American Journal of Infection Control reports between 5 and 18% of patients in an extended care facility will have an active infection. It is easy to understand then why handwashing is such an important part of work practice control. Figure 6.1 shows the recommended technique for effective handwashing. Hands should always be washed for the following occasions:

- Before putting on and after removing gloves
- Before and after any patient care not requiring gloves
- Whenever hands are soiled

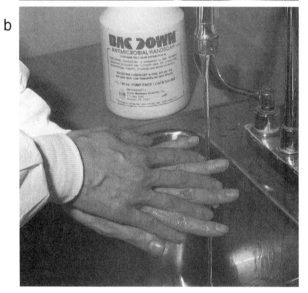

FIGURE 6.1

a. First palm to palm.

b. Next, the palm of one hand over the back of the other hand. Repeat the procedure reversing hands.

c. Now wash hands palm to palm with fingers interlaced.

d. Wash back of fingers of one hand against the palm of the other hand. Repeat reversing hands.

e. Rotate the thumb in the palm. Again repeat reversing hands.

f. Last, rotate the fingers of each hand in the palm of the other.

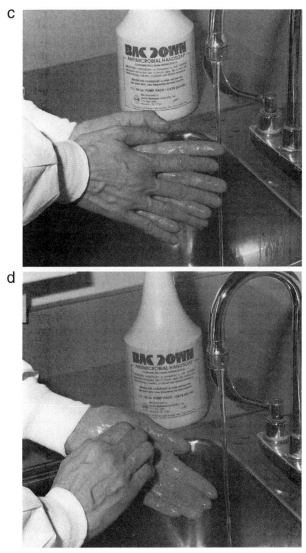

FIGURE 6 1—*continued*

e

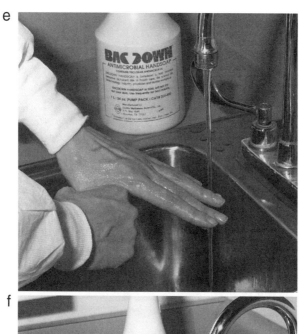

f

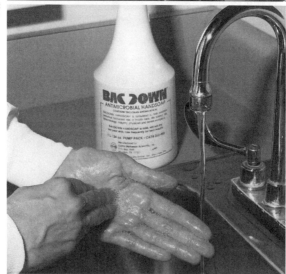

FIGURE 6.1—*continued*

- After wiping or blowing your nose
- After going to the toilet
- Before eating or drinking
- After any cleaning activity
- Before leaving the work area

PERSONAL PROTECTIVE EQUIPMENT

Employers must require employees who may be exposed to blood borne pathogens to use appropriate **PPE.** All PPE must be supplied at the employer's expense. Although this may include a variety of different items, our discussion will be limited to gloves, gowns, and face protectors. The selection of PPE depends on the nature of the exposure. Rules to follow for all PPE include:

- Always wear PPE when there is a possibility of exposure to blood borne pathogens.
- Remove and replace PPE that are torn or punctured or has lost the ability to function as a barrier to blood borne pathogens.
- Be sure to remove PPE before leaving work area.

The Role of Gloves in Infection Control

Although unbroken skin is an excellent barrier against disease-causing organisms, unseen microscopic tears and breaks in the hand's skin surface make it more probable that pathogens may infect the bloodstream unless gloves are worn as a protective cover. Gloves should be made of latex, nitryl, rubber, or some other water-impervious material. Gloves are available with and without powder. If an allergic reaction to a particular type of glove is noticed, request another type. Liners for gloves are available. Also, if you know of a cut or abrasion on your hands, it is best to cover it with a plastic adhesive pressure strip or similar protection before putting on the gloves. This adds an additional layer of protection against accidental contamination.

REMOVAL AND DISCARDING OF CONTAMINATED GLOVES
After you have completed a task that requires the use of gloves, remove and dispose of them properly. Figures 6.2 through 6.4 demonstrate the proper removal of contaminated gloves. *Always* discard the gloves in a biohazardous waste container; *never* in a regular trash container. Contaminated gloves discarded in this manner expose others to unexpected biohazards.

QUALITY CONTROL
If the purpose for wearing gloves is to be accomplished, it is paramount that they be fully intact. It is important that before using a pair of gloves you vi-

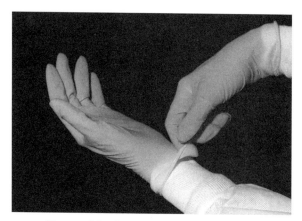

FIGURE 6.2 Grasp the first glove at the wrist.

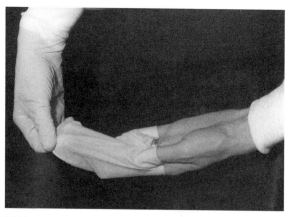

FIGURE 6.3 Fold it over at the wrist and peel back toward the fingers, turning it inside out as it is being removed. Once the glove is off, hold it in the gloved hand.

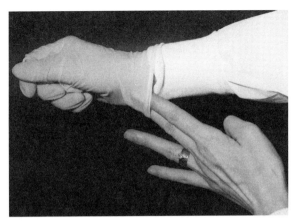

FIGURE 6.4   To remove the other glove, place bare fingers inside the cuff of the glove. Make sure not to touch the exterior of the glove. Remove this glove in a similar manner as the first. It will then envelope the other glove.

sually inspect for gross abnormalities such as tears and holes. Unfortunately, because of the natural elasticity of the gloves, small holes may go unobserved. Most manufacturers test their gloves to make sure the gloves do not have holes. Nevertheless, in addition to visual inspection, you may wish to statistically sample your stock of gloves to confirm the integrity purported by the manufacturer. Two rather simple quality control methods are air and water inflation. However, neither method is foolproof. During air inflation, the glove is inflated on an air jet and visually inspected for holes and escaping air. During water inflation, the glove is filled with water and inspected for leaks. *Remember. If a glove is damaged, don't use it!*

Gowns and Face Protection

Gowns or laboratory coats must be worn to prevent contamination of clothing and protect the skin from blood and body fluid exposure. Gowns and laboratory coats may be disposable or the type that can be sent to a laundry. The degree of impermeability of gowns and laboratory coats depends on the anticipated amount of splashes or quantity of infective material present, and the sleeves should be cuffed at the wrist (Fig. 6.5). Gowns and laboratory coats should always be worn closed. When they become contaminated, they should be removed at the location of use and immediately placed in bags or containers that are clearly marked with a biohazard symbol or color-coded. If potentially infectious materials seep through the gown or laboratory coat and contaminate clothing underneath, these too should be removed as soon as possible and placed in an appropriate bag or container until disposed of or laundered. Any exposed skin should be thoroughly washed with soap and water.

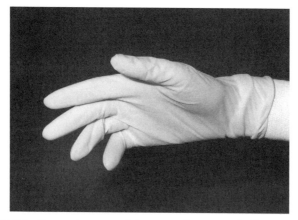

FIGURE 6.5 Proper placement of glove extending over cuff of laboratory coat.

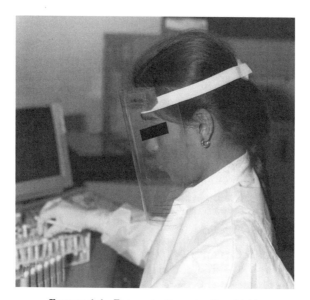

FIGURE 6.6 Face protection using face shield.

When performing procedures where splashing of the face is likely to occur, face protection should also be worn in addition to a gown or laboratory coat. This is to protect the mucous membranes of the eyes, mouth, and nose. Face protection can be a face shield (Fig. 6.6) or glasses or goggles and mask as demonstrated in Figure 6.7. If glasses or goggles are worn, then a mask must also be worn. In certain situations non-PPE safety shields, as shown in Figure 6.8, may be used in lieu of PPE that must be worn.

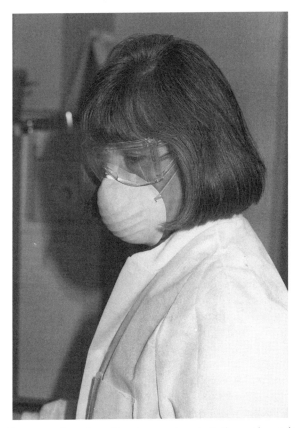

FIGURE 6.7 Face protection using safety glasses and mask. Both must be used together for effective protection.

DECONTAMINATION AND DISINFECTION OF BIOLOGICAL SPILLS

Accidents happen, and it is important for health care employees to be familiar with the proper course of action to follow in ensuring that exposure to infectious materials is minimized. During any decontamination and disinfection procedure, always remember to wear appropriate PPE. Remember too that every accident is different and suitable corrective measures and priorities must be evaluated in each situation. Listed below are suggested steps that may be used for most biological spills.

1. Warn fellow employees in the area of the spill.
2. If present, carefully remove any broken glass using tweezers or a scoop such as ridged cardboard. *Do not use your hands!* Dispose the broken glass in a puncture-proof biohazard receptacle.

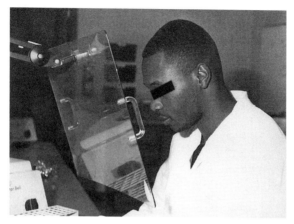

FIGURE 6.8   Photograph showing correct use of a safety shield.

3. Absorb the spilled blood or body fluid by covering with disposable towels. If the spill is large, you may also want to flood the area with a disinfectant by gently pouring a fresh 1:10 or 1:100 solution of 5.25% bleach (sodium hypochlorite) or some other suitable disinfectant on the paper towels.
4. Remove the disposable towels, and clean the area using a detergent.
5. Even if done previously, disinfect the spill site by gently flooding the area with a disinfectant or wiping down the area using disposable towels soaked in a disinfectant.
6. Wipe the area using dry disposable towels or let air dry.
7. Be sure to place all disposable towels in an appropriate biohazard container, remove gloves, and wash hands.

If an accident occurs while centrifuging, interrupt the power to the centrifuge, wait until the centrifuge head comes to a complete halt, then carefully open the safety top. Disinfect according to the manufacturer's recommendations or the written policy of your institution. Work areas should also be wiped down with a suitable disinfectant at the end of each work shift not just when there has been a biological spill.

SHARPS AND OTHER BIOHAZARDOUS WASTE DISPOSAL

A far too common occurrence is the injury of health care employees by improperly disposed needles and broken glass. A needle carelessly left in a bed or broken glass poking through a garbage bag may injure and needlessly expose employees to infectious material that may have been on the needle or broken glass. It cannot be stressed strongly enough that it is important to handle and dispose of sharps in a safe manner. Outlined below are several work practice controls regarding needles and broken glass.

Needles

1. *Do not* hand recap, bend, shear, or break contaminated needles.
2. If for some reason the medical procedure requires that the needle be recapped manually, do so by using a mechanical means such as forceps or the one-handed scoop method.
3. Dispose of contaminated needles in a closable, puncture-resistant, leak-proof container (Fig. 6.9). The container should be constructed as to allow removal of the needle using only one hand. It should also be red in color or have a biohazard symbol prominently displayed. Make sure that containers stay in an upright position and *never* overfill.

Broken Glass

1. *Never* pick up broken glass with your hands.
2. Remove any broken glass using tweezers or *carefully* scoop the broken glass into a dustpan or something equally suitable using a ridged object such as cardboard.
3. Dispose of all broken glass in a closable, puncture-resistant container. Containers into which contaminated glassware has been disposed should conspicuously display a biohazard symbol.

Biohazardous Waste

In addition to sharps and gloves, items such as gauze, plastic pressure bandages, or disposable towels that are used for cleaning and are caked with dried

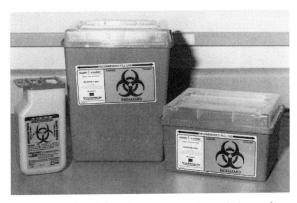

FIGURE 6.9   Examples of closable, puncture-resistant, leak-proof containers.

blood or have come in contact with potentially infectious materials and all body fluids, pathological tissues, and microbiological refuse are considered biological waste and must be placed in appropriate containers that are colored red and, if labeled, display the universal biohazard symbol (Fig. 6.10) to warn of their contents. Laws governing the disposal of medical waste vary from state to state. Some states require that only licensed medical waste disposal facilities collect and dispose of biohazardous material.

TRAINING

OSHA's Blood Borne Pathogen Standard 29 CFR 1910.1030 mandates that employees be trained initially upon their job assignment. Additional training may be needed if the employee is reassigned to another position or given added responsibilities. Updates should be given annually. The individual doing the training must be knowledgeable about the material to be covered and must present it in a manner appropriate in content & vocabulary to the educational level, literacy, and language of the employees being trained. During the training, ample time must be allowed for questions and answers. A copy of the OSHA's standard must be available, and the training should be tailored for the job assignment and must include discussion of blood borne diseases and their transmission, the facilities' exposure control plan, work practice controls, response to exposure incidents (including post-exposure and follow-up), and the availability of hepatitis B vaccine.

HEPATITIS B VACCINE

OSHA Blood Borne Pathogens Standard requires that employees who may have occupational exposure to blood contaminated with hepatitis B be offered the hepatitis B vaccine. The vaccine must be made available to the employee at no cost, at a reasonable time and location, and within 10 working days after the employee has accepted the job assignment. The vaccine must be administered under the supervision of a licensed health care professional and given according to the latest guidelines of the United States Public Health Service. Prescreen-

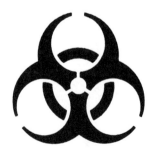

FIGURE 6.10   Biohazard symbol.

ing cannot be a prerequisite for receiving the vaccine. If an employee chooses not to take the vaccine, the employee must sign a declination form. However, if at a later date the employee decides to take the vaccine, it must be given at no cost. There are several reasons why an employee should not receive the vaccine. These include: 1) previously completing the hepatitis B vaccination series, 2) laboratory testing indicates the employee is already immune to hepatitis B, and 3) there are medical contraindications for receiving the vaccine.

ENGINEERING CONTROLS

Work practice controls are those procedures that health care employees must follow on the job to reduce exposure to blood borne diseases and other infectious materials. These include the wearing of face protection, gowns, gloves; proper disposal of needles and biohazardous waste; and the washing of hands. Engineering controls are physical or mechanical systems that attempt to eliminate hazards at their source. They may, in some instances, alter the work practice. For example, work shields as shown in Figure 6.8 can be used in work areas where there are anticipated splashes or sprays, thus eliminating the need to wear a mask and eye protection.

Each year nearly 800,000 health care professionals are exposed to infectious blood because of needle sticks. In the past few years a number of biomedical companies have developed products that may be used as engineering controls to help reduce needle stick injuries. A few representatives include a needle that self-blunts prior to removal from the patient, a one-handed closing technique that locks a shield over the needle point immediately after withdrawal from the patient, and needle adapters that slide and lock in place over the needle after use. In addition to engineering controls against needle sticks, there are single-use lancing devices that automatically retract, thus helping eliminate potential sticks after doing capillary punctures. Shatterproof blood collection tubes are another example of an engineering control developed to help prevent exposure to blood borne infections. It is important to remember, however, that the effectiveness of any engineering control depends on its proper use by the health care worker.

Body Substance Isolation and HICPAC Isolation Precautions

The first published recommendations for isolation precautions in the United States appeared in a hospital handbook in 1877. Between that date and 1970, a number of different infectious control practices were recommended. Then, in 1970, the CDC published a detailed manual entitled "Isolation Techniques for Use in Hospitals." It was the first serious attempt to standardize isolation practices that could be applied to both small and large hospitals. The manual introduced the category system of isolation precautions. There were seven: Strict Isolation, Respiratory Isolation, Protective Isolation, Enteric Precautions, Wound and Skin Precautions, Discharge Precautions, and Blood Precautions. The precautions recommended for each of the categories were primarily determined by their routes of transmission.

With the introduction of UP in 1985 and the OSHA Blood-Borne Pathogens Rule in 1989, it became obvious that no single system could address all the isolation precaution needs of the more than 6,000 hospitals in the United States. In December 1995, the Hospital Infection Control Practices Advisory Committee (HICPAC) published their recommendations for isolation precautions in hospitals.

The HICPAC isolation precautions has two tiers. The first tier, which is the most important, is called **Standard Precautions** (Fig. 6.11). It synthesizes the major features of the OSHA Blood-Borne Pathogens Rule and UP. Standard precautions are applied to all patients receiving hospital care regardless of their diagnosis or presumed infectious status. The primary goal of standard precautions is the successful control of nosocomial infections. The second tier includes precautions designed for patients known or suspected to be infected with epidemiologically important pathogens that can be transmitted by direct or indirect contact. This second tier is known as **Transmission-Based Precautions.** There are three types of transmission-based precautions: airborne, droplet, and contact. The precautions may be used singularly or in combination, and they must be used *in addition to* the standard precautions. For patients for whom transmission-based precautions are necessary, color coded signs with a synopsis of the precautions printed on them may be placed on the door of the patient's room (Figs. 6.12 to 6.14). The precautions are to be read and followed explicitly. Some hospitals prefer to affix a stop sign to the door such as the one illustrated in Figure 6.15. If such a sign is used, health care employees and visitors must report to the nurses' desk for instructions regarding any special precautions before entering the patient's room.

CHEMICAL HAZARDS

In 1988, OSHA introduced the **Hazard Communication Standard,** also know as the "Right-to-Know Rule." This regulation was implemented to prevent adverse effects to employees from chemical hazards. The discussions below focus on workplace programs that, if implemented, will help prevent the occurrence of work-related illnesses and injuries caused by chemicals.

Material Safety Data Sheets

Material Safety Data Sheets (MSDS) are the backbone of any chemical safety program. OSHA requires chemical manufacturers to make available an

STANDARD PRECAUTIONS
(For use on all patients)

Handwashing
1. Wash hands after touching blood, body fluids, secretions, excretions, and and contaminated items.
2. Wash hands immediately after gloves are removed and between patient contact to avoid transfer of microorganisms to other patients or environments

Gloves
1. Wear gloves in situations when you may be exposed to blood, body fluids, secretions, excretions, and contaminated items
2. Put on clean gloves just before touching mucous membranes and nonintact skin.
3. Change gloves between tasks and procedures on the same patient after contact with material that may contain high concentrations of microorganisms.
4. Remove gloves promptly after use and properly dispose in a biohazard container identified for such purposes.

Eye, Nose, and Mouth Protection
Protect mucous membranes of the eyes, nose, and mouth with mask and eye protection or face shield when doing procedures and patient-care activities that are likely to generate splashes or sprays of blood, body fluids, secretions, or excretions

Gowning
1. Put on gown when it is necessary to protect skin and prevent soiling of clothing during procedures that are likely to generate splashes or sprays of blood, body fluids, secretions, or excretions.
2. Remove a soiled gown as promptly as possible and properly dispose in a biohazard container identified for such purposes.

Patient-Care Equipment
Handle used patient-care equipment soiled with blood, body fluids, secretions, or excretions in a manner that prevents exposure to skin. mucous membranes, and clothing. Ensure that reusable equipment is not used for the care of another patient until it has been appropriately cleaned and reprocessed. Use single-use items if at all possible and properly dispose in biohazard containers identified for such purposes.

Environmental Control
Follow health care facility procedures for routine care, cleaning, and disinfection of environmental surfaces such as beds, bed rails, bedside equipment, and other frequently touched surfaces.

FIGURE 6.11   HICPAC Standard Precautions.

AIRBORNE PRECAUTIONS
(In addition to Standard Precautions)

Patient Placement
1. Use private room that has a) monitored negative air pressure, b) six to twelve air exchanges per hour, and c) discharge of air outdoors or if room air recirculated, HEPA filtration.
2. Keep room door closed and patient must remain in room.

Respiratory Protection
1. Wear N95 respirator when entering the room of a patient with known or suspected infectious pulmonary tuberculosis.
2. Susceptible persons should not enter room of patients known or suspected to have measles (rubeola) or varicella (chickenpox). If susceptible persons must enter the room, they should wear N95 respirator.
3. Respirators are not required if immune to measles or varicella.

Patient Transport
1. Limit transport of patient to essential purposes only.
2. Use surgical mask on patient during transport.

Visitors
Report to nurses' station before entering room.

FIGURE 6.12   HICPAC Airborne Precautions.

DROPLET PRECAUTIONS
(In addition to Standard Precautions)

Patient Placement
Private room, if possible; maintain spatial separation of three feet from other patients if private room is not available

Mask
Wear mask when working within three feet of patient or upon entering room.

Patient Transport
1. Limit transport of patient from room to essential purposes only.
2. Use mask on patient during transport.

Visitors
Report to nurses' station before entering room.

FIGURE 6.13   HICPAC Droplet Precautions.

CONTACT PRECAUTIONS
(In addition to Standard Precautions)

Patient Placement
Private room, if possible; may cohort if private room is not available

Gloves
1. Wear gloves when entering patient room.
2. Change gloves after having contact with infective material that may contain high concentrations of microorganisms (fecal material and wound drainage).
3. Remove gloves before leaving patient's room. Wash hands after gloves are removed. Properly dispose of gloves in a biohazard container identified for such purposes.

Handwashing
Wash hands with an antimicrobial agent immediately after glove removal. After glove removal and handwashing, ensure that hands do not touch potentially contaminated environmental surfaces or items in the patient's room to avoid transfer of microorganisms to other patients or environments.

Gowning
1. Wear gowns when entering patient's room if you anticipate that your clothing will have substantial contact with the patient, environmental surfaces, or items in the patient's room or if the patient is incontinent or has diarrhea, has an ileostomy or colostomy, or wound drainage not contained by a dressing.
2. Remove gown before leaving the patient's environment and ensure that clothing does not contact potentially contaminated environmental surfaces to avoid transfer of microorganisms to other patients or environments. Place gown in a biohazard container identified for such purposes.

Patient Transport
Limit transport of patients to essential purposes only. During transport, ensure that precautions are maintained to minimize the risk of transmission of microorganisms to other patients and contamination of environmental surfaces and equipment.

Patient-Care Equipment
1. Dedicate the use of noncritical patient-care equipment to a single patient.
2. If common equipment is used, clean and disinfect between patients.

Visitors
Report to nurses' station before entering room.

FIGURE 6.14   HICPAC Contact Precautions.

REPORT TO NURSE
BEFORE ENTERING

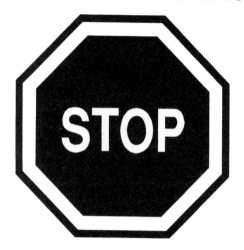

**FAVOR DE ANUNCIARSE A LA ENFERMERA DE PISO
ANTES DE ENTRAR AL CUARTO**

FIGURE 6.15   Stop sign that may be used in lieu of printed precautions (Courtesy of Briggs Corporation, 800-247-2343).

MSDS for each hazardous chemical they manufacture or import. The MSDS contains more detailed information than that listed on the label attached to the individual chemical container. The MSDS provides more detailed information regarding special conditions for safe handling and properties of the chemical than the label attached to the chemical container. While the employer must make the MSDS available during working hours, it is the responsibility of the employee to know where the MSDS is located and to apply good professional judgment to the information it contains. It is a good idea when working with a new chemical to review its MSDS in order to familiarize oneself with any hazards or precautions that should be taken when working with the new chemical. Not all MSDS look alike, but they must all include the following information:

• Identity of the substance on the container label
• Name, address, and telephone number for hazard and emergency information.
• Date the MSDS was prepared
• Chemical and common names of hazardous ingredients found in the product

- Permissible exposure limits
- Physical and chemical characteristics of the product, such as appearance, odor, boiling point, and vapor pressure
- Physical hazards, including the potential for fire, explosion, and reactivity and the proper extinguishing media
- Primary routes of entry into the body (e.g., ingestion, inhalation, and skin absorption)
- Acute and chronic health hazards, including signs and symptoms of exposure and medical conditions aggravated by exposure
- Carcinogenic hazard characteristics
- Emergency and first aid procedures
- Safe handling procedures, including work practice, spill or leak cleanup, storage and transport precautions, and protective measures for maintenance
- Appropriate waste disposal

Warning and Safety Symbols

In addition to the biohazard symbol discussed earlier, there are a number of other important symbols with which health care workers need to be familiar. Several of the more common are discussed below.

POISON, TOXIC, OR IRRITANT HAZARD

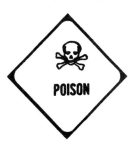

The black and white symbol of a skull and crossbones indicates the presence of a poisonous, toxic, or irritant agent. In addition to proper safety techniques, protective barriers should be worn and safety equipment should be in use when handling these agents. It is also important to be knowledgeable regarding OSHA's allowable safe exposure limits for the particular agent being used. These limits are called threshold limit values (TLVs), and they may be located in the MSDS on each agent. The proper emergency and first aid procedures in case of an accident will also be included in the MSDS. At the bottom of the sign is a number. This number is a code that identifies the type of hazard to which the chemical is classified. For example, the number 5.1 at the bottom of a sign indicates that it is an oxidizer.

Table 6.1 lists the hazard classes.

CORROSIVE HAZARD

Corrosive agents include such chemicals as sulfuric acid, hydrochloric acid, and sodium hydroxide. These agents can cause harmful injury to the skin, eyes, and respiratory tract. Proper safety techniques should include the wear-

TABLE 6.1. THE DEPARTMENT OF TRANSPORTATION HAZARD CLASSES

Hazard Class	DOT Hazard Class ID Number
Igniters (e.g., explosives)	1
Gases (i.e., non-flammable, flammable, poison/toxic)	2
Flammable liquids	3
Flammable solids	4
Oxidizer/organic peroxide	5
Poison/toxic (e.g., infectious substances)	6
Radioactive	7
Corrosive	8
Miscellaneous dangerous goods	9

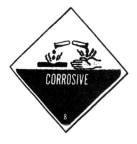

ing of protective barriers. In case of accidental contact with corrosive chemicals, the affected area should be flooded with copious amounts of water. Chemical splashes to the eyes pose special physical requirements. The Code of Federal Regulations 1910.151(c) notes that when the eyes of any person may be exposed to corrosive chemicals, the employer will provide within the work area a suitable facility for quick flushing of the eyes. General requirements are that the eyewash can be turned on in 1 second or less with both eyes closed, it will flush both eyes simultaneously, it must have a "stay open" feature so that both hands can be free to open the eyelids, and it can deliver a stream of water at no less than 0.4 gallons per minute for 15 minutes.

RADIATION HAZARD

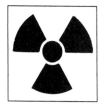

This symbol for radiation hazard is usually red on a yellow or white background. It indicates that some type of radioactive material is in the vicinity. Safety procedures depend on the level of possible exposure. Safety procedures may require the use of lead shielding upon exposure to x-rays or wearing gloves when performing a laboratory procedure that uses a minimal amount of radioactive material. Health care professionals involved in any procedure using radioactive material should make themselves knowledgeable regarding their institution's policies on radiation exposure, spills, and contamination.

FLAMMABLE HAZARD

The warning sign for flammable agents may use a variety of backgrounds. Common to all, however, is the distinctive symbolic flame. Flammable liquids are defined as liquids that are readily ignitable at room temperature. The Department of Transportation and the National Fire Protection Association (NFPA) further define flammable liquids as a liquid with a flash point below 100° F (38° C). A **flash point** is the temperature at which a liquid gives off enough vapor to ignite. Ethyl alcohol, toluene, and xylene are examples of flammable agents that may be used by health care workers. When used in small quantities, flammable agents should be stored in approved safety containers and placed in safety storage cabinets. They are *never* to be used near sources of ignition such as open flames, heaters, or sparking motors.

The National Fire Protection Association Chemical Hazard Sign

The NFPA uses a symbol system designed in a diamond shape, which contains four different colored diamonds. A number from 0 to 4 is placed in each diamond to indicate the order of severity. Below is an explanation of what each color represents and its number coding system.

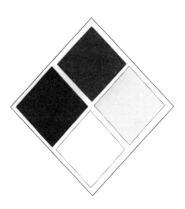

Blue Diamond—Health Hazard

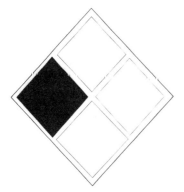

4: Deadly
3: Extreme Danger
2: Hazardous
1: Slightly Hazardous
0: Normal Material

RED DIAMOND—FLAMMABILITY

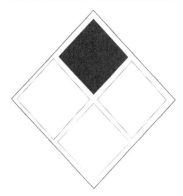

4: Flash point below 73° F
3: Flash point below 100° F
2: Flash point above 100° F, not exceeding 200° F
1: Flash point above 200° F
0: Will not burn

YELLOW DIAMOND—REACTIVITY

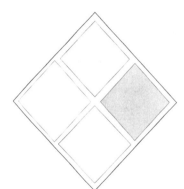

4: May detonate
3: Shock and heat may detonate
2: Violent chemical change
1: Unstable if heated
0: Stable

WHITE DIAMOND—SPECIAL HAZARDS

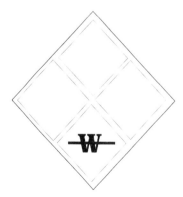

OX: Oxidizer
ACID: Acid
ALK: Alkali
CORR: Corrosive
W̶:   Use NO WATER
P: Polymerization

The NFPA label illustrated below is for acetone. Note that it may be slightly hazardous to health, it is a flammable liquid since it has a flash point below 100° F, it is stable, and there are no special hazards that must be noted.

Proper Handling and Disposal of Chemicals

When hazardous chemicals are improperly handled, stored, or disposed, serious problems may result, including personal injury, fire, corrosion, damage to sewage systems, environmental pollution, and even explosions. It is vitally important that all chemicals be handled in a safe manner and disposed of appropriately. The health care employee should be knowledgeable about all chemicals being used and follow the recommendations on each as described in the MSDS. In addition to the safe handling practices discussed elsewhere in this chapter, it is stressed here to remember that 1) all containers should be clearly labeled, noting the name of the chemical and listing the hazards that may result in their use, 2) make sure to read all labels before using a chemical, 3) use only the amount of chemical that is needed, 4) handle chemical containers carefully in order to minimize the chance of accidents, and 5) when through using a chemical, make sure the opening is securely closed and the chemical stored correctly. Knowledge regarding the proper disposal of excess or outdated chemicals is just as important as proficiency in their use and storage. Instructions on disposal for each chemical are found under Section VII of the MSDS. Regardless, be sure to check with local and state agencies about their chemical disposal guidelines. Some water soluble chemicals may be disposed in the laboratory sink by flushing with large amounts of water. Others may need to be disposed of by a licensed chemical disposal company.

Chemical Spills

All chemicals should be treated as hazardous, so in the event of a chemical spill, the following general steps should be taken:

1. All employees in the vicinity of the spill should be notified and evacuated if necessary. The immediate supervisor should also be alerted.
2. If necessary, make sure there is proper ventilation.
3. Review the MSDS on the chemical to see if any special precautions need to be taken.
4. Put on heavy chemical-resistant rubber gloves and other appropriate protective wear.
5. If broken glass is present, using tongs, carefully remove and dispose of the broken glass into a puncture-proof–leak-proof container.
6. If a commercial spill kit is available, open, and follow instructions. If a spill kit is not available, cover the spill with an appropriate neutralizing agent such as sodium bicarbonate or dry soda ash.
7. Absorb the liquid using a vermiculite or a large number of paper towels.
8. Carefully place absorption materials into containers identified for this purpose, and put them in the designated location for pick up and final disposition.
9. Clean the area with soap and water. Dry.

EMERGENCY AND FIRE SAFETY

Fortunately, few fires are encountered in health care facilities, but the potential exists. When fires occur, the most frequent causes are carelessness because of complacency, faulty electronic equipment or wiring, unattended operations, and lack of personnel training. Following is a general list of some of the fire safety and emergency precautions that should be observed by all health care employees.

* Know the locations and types of fire extinguishers (A, B, C) in your facility. Know how to use them and on what kinds of fires each type may be used.
  On some fire extinguishers you may notice numbers preceding the letters. These numbers indicate the extinguishers' relative effectiveness in extinguishing that class of fire. For example, a fire extinguisher with a 3A-40 BC rating is suppose to be four times as effective in putting out combustible liquid and electrical fires as an extinguisher with a 3A-10 BC rating. Bear in mind that these ratings are made under controlled laboratory conditions, which may not mimic real-life situations.

To effectively operate an extinguisher, think P-A-S-S
  •P—pull the pin
  •A—aim the hose at the base of the fire
  •S—squeeze the handle
  •S—sweep the hose back and forth

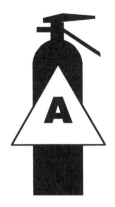 For fires involving wood, paper, and clothing. Employs water or an all-purpose dry chemical.

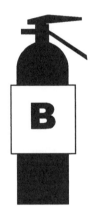 For fires involving flammable liquid or gases. Employs foam, dry chemical or carbon dioxide.

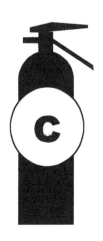 For fires near or in electrical equipment. Employs an extinguishing agent that will not conduct electricity such as carbon dioxide or some other dry chemical.

- Be familiar with the fire alert system, the fire escape plan, and how to report a fire in your health care facility. RACE for safety.

RESCUE patients	Activate an **ALARM** or call our fire code
CONFINE the blaze	**EXTINGUISH** fire if small, otherwise **EVACUATE**

- Have all fire extinguishers inspected at least every 12 months for broken seals, damages, low gauge pressure, or improper mounting.
- Know the location of all circuit breakers or master switches in your facility or work area. Know what to do if a fellow employee is electrocuted.
- Store flammable agents in explosion-proof cabinets or refrigerators.
- As part of a preventive maintenance program, conduct and document annual safety checks on electrical equipment.
- Annually check the grounding and polarity on all electrical outlets.
- Establish an employee safety training program, and annually hold a fire evacuation drill.

PAY ATTENTION TO ERGONOMICS

The word ergonomics comes from a combination of the Greek word *ergo,* which means "work," and *nomics,* which means "study." Ergonomics then is the study of the capacities and requirements of workers and their interaction with the equipment they use, their work process, and the environment in which they work. In other words, ergonomics means fitting the workplace to the worker by modifying or redesigning the job, work area, equipment, or environment. The scope or purpose of ergonomics is to minimize employee exposure to hazards that lead to **cumulative trauma disorders** (CTDs). OSHA will soon publish ergonomic standards for all workplaces.

Cumulative Trauma Disorders

RISK FACTORS

CTD is a group of health problems that involve soft tissue such as muscles, tendons, joints, and nerves. All CTDs have similar characteristics and are caused by wear and tear from repetitive motion. Some of the risk factors associated with CTD include:

- Tasks that require high repetition
- Excessive physical strength required for the task
- Poor posture and movement of the limbs and body as a task is performed
- Poor design of work area or equipment

COMMON CUMULATIVE TRAUMA DISORDERS

Disorder	Symptoms	Cause	Occurrence
Tendonitis	Pain, swelling, and tenderness in hand, elbow, or shoulder	Inflammation of tendon in hand and wrist because of excessive use	Phlebotomists
Tendosynovitis	Pain, swelling, and tenderness in hand or arm	Inflammation of tendon and sheath surrounding tendon because of excessive use.	Phlebotomists
Trigger Finger	Snapping and jerking movement when attempting to move finger	Tendon sheath is swollen-tendon and becomes locked in sheath because of groove in flexing tendon	Histopathology laboratory workers
Carpal Tunnel Syndrome (CTS)	Pain, numbness, tingling, and loss of strength in hand; sometimes paralysis	Compression or pinching of median nerve that runs through wrist because of poor work area design	Healthcare workers involved in data entry, transcription, and tedious laboratory procedures
Back Disorders	Sharp or nagging pain	Pinched nerves because of inflamed muscles, which are caused by bending, reaching, carrying, lifting, or moving loads that are too heavy or big	Healthcare workers

- Temperature too cold
- Holding a position for prolonged periods

COMMON CUMULATIVE TRAUMA DISORDERS

Prevention

Prevention is the key to reducing or eliminating the risk of developing CTD. Although much of the burden rests with the employer to make sure that a good ergonomic program is in place, no amount of effort to reduce or eliminate CTD risk can be accomplished unless employees are willing to do their part. Below are several preventive measures that employees can do on their own.

1. Use good body posture when sitting. Select the right chair for the job to be done.
2. Preventive measures for personnel performing computer tasks:
   a) The computer monitor should be directly in front and at a viewing distance of 18 to 24 inches (45 to 60 cm) from the eyes. The display screen should be at or slightly below eye level. Make sure the display screen is clean in order to maintain character clarity and reduce the reflection of light.
   b) The keyboard should also be directly in front and at approximately elbow height. Use a wrist rest for support and to help maintain a neutral wrist position (Fig. 6.16).
   c) When using an input device such as a mouse, locate it near the keyboard and use the whole arm to move it instead of just the wrist. Keep it at a natural elevation—not reaching forward or raising the shoulder.
3. If the feet cannot comfortably reach the floor when you are sitting, use a footrest. The footrest should be adjustable and have a heel stop.
4. Once each hour or as needed the following exercises should be performed:
   a) Eyes: roll, palm, and look away
   b) Head and neck: roll head, turn head from side to side, and yawn
   c) Shoulders: Shrug, squeeze, and roll
   d) Back: Stretch upward and reach out
   e) Arms: reach arms in outward position and rotate
   f) Wrist and hands: stretch, rotate, and shake
   g) Feet: stretch
5. Use PPE such as back braces, anti-fatigue mats, anti-glare screens, and wrist braces. A word of caution, do not wear a wrist brace without a physician's order. By doing so, it could be fitted wrong and make things worse.
6. To minimize the risk of developing back injury, use proper lifting techniques. If at all possible, supplies should be stored above knee height and below shoulder height. Lift and carry heavy loads with two hands rather than one, and avoid manipulating loads or objects alone that are too

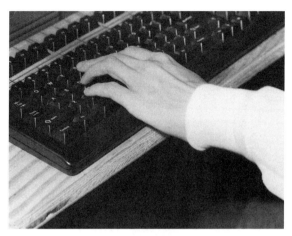

FIGURE 6.16   Illustration showing the position of a neutral wrist.

heavy or large. Always get assistance when needed. There are no legal maximum weight limits that can be lifted by employees, but the National Institute for Occupational Safety recommends a maximum of 51 pounds (23 kg).

7. Generally, the optimum work height for standing or sitting should be done at approximately elbow height. Work should be adjusted to that height if possible. For tasks that have extensive vision requirements such as using the microscope, the work height should be increased as demonstrated in Figure 6.17.

It is important to prevent CTD because musculoskeletal disorders are one of the leading causes of disability among workers and result in suffering and decreased productivity.

GENERAL RULES FOR SAFETY

Several general rules of safety that cannot be easily categorized are listed below. The order in which they are listed has no significance. Although it would be admirable if one could remember and observe each item on this list and the other lists in this chapter, it cannot be emphasized enough that it is important that *each health care employee read and become familiar with the established safety procedure manual for their own health care facility.*

- *Never* eat, smoke, or drink in the laboratory.
- Do not store food or beverages in laboratory refrigerators for specimen or reagent storage.

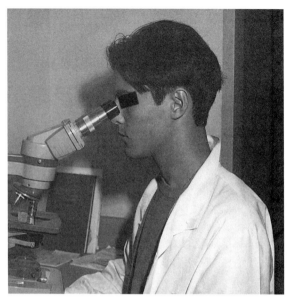

FIGURE 6.17 Note that the microscope is elevated and slightly tilted so that the microscopist does not have to bend and the microscopist's head, neck, and back are reasonably straight.

- *Never* pipette specimens or reagents by mouth.
- Develop the habit of keeping the hands away from the mouth and eyes to prevent self-inoculation with infectious agents.
- Only closed-toe, nonskid-sole shoes should be worn to work in order to prevent possible serious injuries from falls, objects accidentally dropped on the feet, and broken glassware.
- Uniforms and work clothes should be neither tightly form-fitting nor floppy. Aside from looking professional, the reasons for this are that clothes that are too tight inhibit movement and clothes that are floppy could become entangled in mechanical equipment.
- Long hair should be secured away from the face, and beards should be neatly trimmed. Long hair (and even long beards) could become entangled in equipment. Contamination of specimens, work areas, and reagents may occur from shedding of long hair and beards.
- Know what procedure to follow if a fellow employee or patient faints or passes out.
- Take a course in at least basic first aid and cardiopulmonary resuscitation (CPR).
- Attend all departmental and institutional in-service programs on fire prevention and safety.

BIBLIOGRAPHY

Accrocco JO, Cinquanti M, eds. Right-to-know pocket guide for laboratory employees. Schenectady, NY: Genium Publishing Corp., 1992.

American association of physician office laboratories news. Ergonomics. 1996;3(2):1.

Ansell Medical. Donning and glove removal. Available at http://www.ansell.com/latex_gloves/what_you_should_know/J/donning_techniques.html. Accessed on June 24, 1997.

Ansell Medical. Testing gloves for holes. Available at http://www.ansell.com/latex_gloves/what_you_should_know/J/testing_for_holes.html. Accessed on June 24, 1997.

Armstrong SE. The cost of needle-stick injuries: the impact of safer medical devices. Nursing Economics 1991;9(6):426.

Association for Professionals in Infection Control and Epidemiology, Inc. Infection control tips on handwashing. Available at http://www.apci.org/html/cons/washtips.html. Accessed on June 24, 1997.

Boater Education Series. Portable fire extinguishers: can you trust your old flame? (Report No. 27). Boat/US Magazine 1997;11(3):12.

Centers for Disease Control. Part II: recommendations for isolation precautions in hospitals. Available at http://www.cdc.gov/ncidod/hip/isolat/isopart2.htm. Accessed on June 24, 1997.

Centers for Disease Control, USDHHS. Guidelines for prevention of transmission of human immunodeficiency virus and hepatitis B virus to health care and public-safety workers. MMWR Morb Mortal Wkly Rep 1989;38(S-6).

Compliance Control. Hand-transmitted infection. Available at http://users.aol.com/comcontrol/cci2.htm. Accessed on June 24, 1997.

Cummings MJ, Lynch P. Body substance isolation: APIC infection control and applied epidemiology principles and procedures. St. Louis, MO: Mosby, 1996.

Federal Register. Draft guideline for infection control in health care personnel. September 8, 1997;62(173):47476.

Garner JS. Overview of isolation systems: APIC infection control and applied epidemiology principles and procedures. St. Louis, MO: Mosby, 1996.

Giles TJ. What's new in laboratory safety? It's not just OSHA anymore! St. Louis, MO: Giles and Associates, 1994.

Hall L. Blood borne pathogen. Supervisors' update no. 96–09. Available at http://www.eig.com/ssu9605.htm. Accessed on June 28, 1997.

Hospital Infection Control Practices Advisory Committee (HICPAC). Appendix C: Recommendations for isolation precautions in hospitals. APIC infection control and applied epidemiology principles and procedures. St. Louis, MO: Mosby, 1996.

Jagger J, Bentley M. Clinical laboratories: reducing exposure to blood borne pathogens. Advances in Exposure Prevention 1996;2(3):1.

Mobley RC, Tinker G, Shaikh AH, Balsden CR. Laboratory safety: the learning laboratorian series. Augusta, GA: Medical College of Georgia, 1989.

National Committee for Clinical Laboratory Standards: Clinical laboratory safety: tentative guideline. Document GP17-T. Villanova, PA: NCCLS, 1994.

Oklahoma State University. PPE, work practices, and engineering controls. Available at http://www.pp.okstate.edu/ehs/modules/bbpppe.htm. Accessed on June 28, 1997.

Ransom WJ. Pay attention to ergonomics. Available at http://www.sddt.com/~columbus/Files/ran950222.html. Accessed on July 29, 1997.

Southern California Phlebotomy Training Co. Gloving. Rockford, MI: Phlebotic, 1997.

Southern California Phlebotomy Training Co. Preventing needle sticks. Rockford, MI: Phlebotic, 1997.

Texas Workforce Commission. OSHA blood borne pathogen rules, OSHA 3131 1994 (Revised). Available at http://hi-tec.twc.State.tx.us/employer/osha3131.htm. Accessed on June 28, 1997.

University of Kentucky. Performance standards: emergency eyewash and shower equipment. Available at http://www.uky.edu/FiscalAffairs/Environmental/ohs/eyewash.html. Accessed on July 18, 1997.

University of Virginia. Chemical labeling. Available at http://www.virginia.edu/~enhealth/L-M-I-T/label-use.html. Accessed on July 18, 1997.

University of Virginia. Eyewash stations. Available at http://www.virginia.edu/~en-health/S-E/eye-wash.html. Accessed on July 18, 1997.

University of Virginia. Fire safety equipment. Available at http://www.virginia.edu/~enhealth/S-E/fse.html. Accessed on July 18, 1997.

U. S. Department of Labor. Occupational safety and health administration. Guidelines for employer compliance (Advisory) 1918.90 App E. Available at http://www.osha-sec.bov/OshStd_data/1918.0090_App_E.html. Accessed on July 1, 1997.

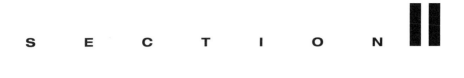

GENERAL PHLEBOTOMY

C H A P T E R **7**

How the Heart and Circulation Work

THE COMPOSITION OF BLOOD

If a tube of blood is allowed to stand undisturbed, it will separate into two major components. One component is red and contains the cellular portion of the blood; the other component is yellowish and can be either clear or hazy in composition. The yellowish component is the liquid portion of the blood. The liquid portion is called either **plasma** or **serum,** depending on whether anticoagulants have been added to the blood sample (Figs 7.1 and 7.2).

Anticoagulants prevent the blood from coagulating or forming a clot. (Anticoagulants and coagulation will be discussed in later sections.) Blood contains a protein substance called **fibrinogen.** Under proper conditions, this substance is converted into another substance called **fibrin.** Fibrin forms a network, which is known as a **clot,** that traps the cellular portion of the blood. The remaining liquid portion is known as **serum.** Because the fibrinogen was converted into fibrin to form to clot, *serum contains no fibrinogen.*

If an anticoagulant is added to the blood, it will not allow the fibrinogen to be converted into fibrin, and no clot will form. Now when the blood sample separates into the two components, the liquid portion is known as **plasma.** *Plasma contains fibrinogen.*

The function of the red blood cells and plasma is to carry oxygen and nourishment to all parts of the body and, at the same time, to pick up waste products from the tissues to be excreted by the kidneys and lungs.

The adult body contains approximately 5 to 6 liters or approximately $1\frac{1}{2}$ gallons of blood. Of this $1\frac{1}{2}$ gallons, approximately 55% is composed of the liquid or fluid portion. The cellular portion of the blood makes up the remaining approximate 45%.

The cellular portion is composed of red blood cells (erythrocytes), white blood cells (leukocytes), and platelets (thrombocytes).

89

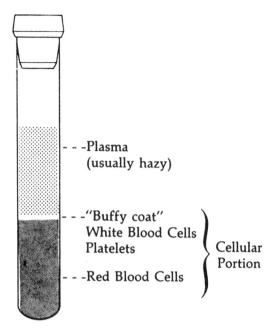

FIGURE 7.1   Anticoagulated blood sample.

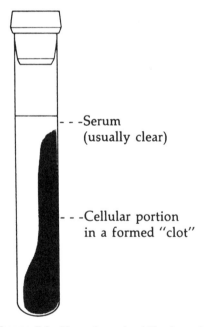

FIGURE 7.2   Nonanticoagulated blood sample.

In general, the red blood cell is a solution of hemoglobin that is contained within a membrane. The life span of a red blood cell is between 100 and 120 days. In the adult, red blood cells are produced in the bone marrow of the axial skeleton and proximal ends of the long bone (Fig. 7.3). The normal red cell is a biconcave disc (Fig. 7.4), which has an average diameter of 7.5 to 8.3 microns (approximately 7/25,000 of an inch).

The white blood cells are produced by the lymph nodes, spleen, thymus, and bone marrow. There are five main types of white blood cells: the neutrophilic series, eosinophilic series, basophilic series, lymphocytic series, and the monocytic series. Examples of the normal mature forms of each series are illustrated in Figure 7.5.

The entire series of white blood cells is designed to defend the body against foreign substances; however, each of the types of cells, neutrophils, monocytes, and the others has a different function. One of the main differences be-

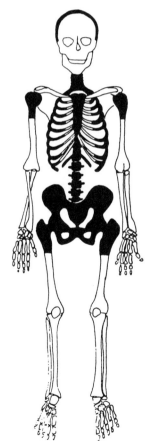

FIGURE 7.3   Red cell marrow distribution in the adult.

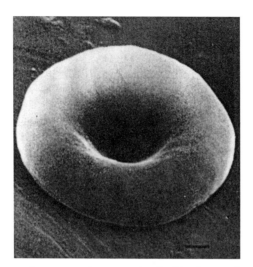

Figure 7.4 The normal mature erythrocyte as visualized by the scanning electron microscope (×9800). (Courtesy of Dr. Wallace N. Jensen from Wintrobe MM, et al. Clinical hematology, 8th ed. Philadelphia, PA: Lea & Febiger, 1981.)

tween red blood cells and white blood cells is that the red cells function intravascularly (i.e., within the veins and capillaries), whereas the white cells function extravascularly (i.e., in the tissues, outside the veins and capillaries). White blood cells simply use the veins and capillaries (the blood) as roads to get from one place to another.

The remaining cellular elements in the blood are the platelets. Platelets function primarily in the stoppage of bleeding. They are produced directly from the cytoplasm of a large cell called the megakaryocyte and have a life span of 9 to 12 days.

THE HEART

The heart is a highly muscular organ, containing four chambers. The two upper chambers are called the **atria;** the two lower chambers are called **ventricles.** The heart is surrounded by a fibrous sac called the **pericardium.** This sac helps to hold the heart in position and isolates it from the other contents of the chest (i.e., thoracic cavity). The inner surfaces and cavities of the heart are lined with a thin but strong membrane called the *endocardium.* If the pericardium becomes inflamed, the condition is called **pericarditis.** Inflammation of the endocardium is referred to as **endocarditis.**

The following outline explains the circulation of the blood through the heart in more detail. Unless instructed otherwise, the reader should refer to the diagram showing the exploded view of the heart (Fig. 7.6).

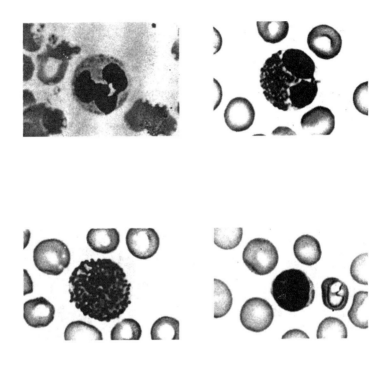

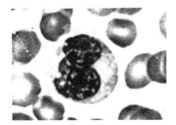

FIGURE 7.5   Photomicrographs of mature white blood cells. (Adapted with permission from Brown BA. Hematology: principles and procedures, 4th ed. Philadelphia, PA: Lea & Febiger, 1984.)

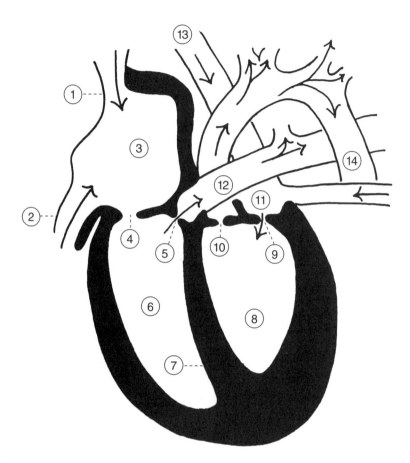

1. Superior Vena Cava
2. Inferior Vena Cava
3. Right Atrium
4. Tricuspid Valve
5. Pulmonary Valve
6. Right Ventricle
7. Septum

8. Left Ventricle
9. Mitral (Bicuspid) Valve
10. Aortic Valve
11. Left Atrium
12. Pulmonary Artery
13. Pulmonary Vein
14. Aorta

FIGURE 7.6 Exploded view of the heart.

1. Returning blood enters the **right atrium** from the **inferior** and **superior vena cava.**
2. The blood then flows from the right atrium through the **tricuspid valve,** filling the **right ventricle.** The tricuspid valve is one of four valves located in the heart. These valves control the direction and flow of blood through the heart.

3. As the right ventricle fills with blood, an electric impulse is delivered, causing the right atrium to contract, thus completing the filling of the right ventricle.
4. The heart initiates its own electric impulses without any stimulation from the brain. The conduction system of the heart is composed of four structures: the **sinoatrial node** (SA node) (also known as the pacemaker), the **atrioventricular node** (AV node), the **AV bundle** or bundle of His, and **Purkinje fibers** (Figure 7.7). These structures are modified cardiac muscles, which differ in function from ordinary cardiac muscles. The initial impulse takes place at the SA node, which is located at the junction of the right atrium and the superior vena cava. The impulse travels first through the atria, causing them to contract. As the impulse reaches the AV node (located in the right atrium near the septum), it slows down a bit so that the atria can completely contract before the ventricles are stimulated. After the electric impulse passes through the AV node, it picks up velocity

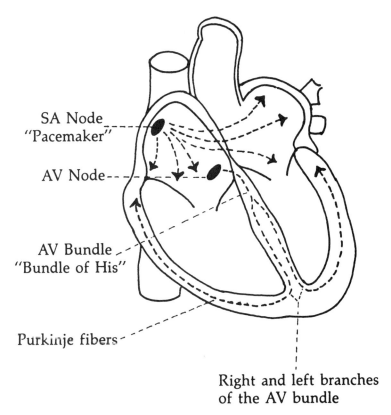

SA Node "Pacemaker"

AV Node

AV Bundle "Bundle of His"

Purkinje fibers

Right and left branches of the AV bundle

FIGURE 7.7   The conduction system of the heart.

as it is relayed through the AV bundle into the ventricles by the Purkinje fibers. This causes the ventricles to contract almost simultaneously. These electric impulses are delivered at precisely timed intervals.

5. In reality, the heart is a double pump. Both sides perform almost simultaneously, sending blood to different places. In other words, when the right atrium contracts, the left atrium contracts at approximately the same time. The same is true for the right and left ventricles. (Fig. 7.8.)

6. When the right ventricle is full, it is stimulated by the electric impulse to begin contraction. As the pressure within the ventricle increases, it causes the tricuspid valve to close. This prevents the blood from flowing backwards into the right atrium.

7. As the ventricular pressure continues to increase, it causes the tricuspid valve to close and forces the blood through the *pulmonary valve* into the *pulmonary artery,* where it flows to the lungs.

8. At the end of the ventricular contraction, the pulmonary valve closes, so that the blood, just expelled, will not flow back into the ventricles.

9. The oxygen-rich blood now returns to the heart through the **pulmonary veins.** These veins empty the blood into the **left atrium.**

10. The blood flows from the left atrium, through the **mitral valve,** filling the **left ventricle.**

11. An electric impulse is delivered from the SA node.

12. The left atrium contracts, thus completing the filling of the left ventricle.

13. When the left ventricle is filled, the electric impulse stimulates the ventricle to begin contraction. As the pressure within the ventricle increases, it causes the mitral valve to close, thus preventing a backward flow of blood into the left atrium.

14. At the same time, this ventricular pressure forces the blood through the **aortic valve** into the **aorta** to circulate throughout the body.

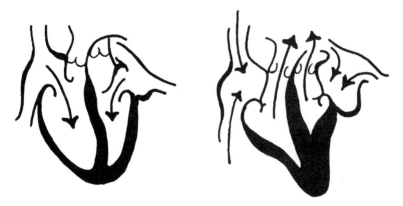

FIGURE 7.8 Diagram illustrating the cardiac cycle. Note that the blood flows from both atria simultaneously and that both ventricles contract at approximately the same time.

15. At the end of the contraction, the aortic valve closes to prevent the back-flow of blood.

The heart is composed of a specialized muscle called the **cardiac muscle.** The muscular wall of the heart is referred to as the **myocardium.** Like other muscles, it contracts and relaxes (approximately 72 times per minute); but unlike other muscles, it never completely rests.

The average weight of the heart is between 250 to 300 grams, and its size is approximately that of an adult fist. Like all other organs in the body, the heart must also have an adequate supply of blood to function properly. Although its chambers are continually filled with blood, the heart cannot directly use this for its own needs. So just like other organs of the body, it receives its blood from the aorta. The first two branches of the aorta (i.e., the left and right coronary arteries) supply the heart with its blood needs. If, for some reason, the smaller arteries branching from the **left** and **right coronary arteries** become closed (i.e., occluded) so that blood cannot pass through, necrosis of the cardiac muscle will occur. This is called a **myocardial infarction** or a heart attack.

VEINS AND ARTERIES
Anatomy

Veins and arteries have walls constructed of three coats (Fig. 7.9). The inner coat, also called the **tunica interna** or **intima,** is composed of (1) simple squamous epithelial cells, which line the lumen of the vessel, (2) a connective tissue layer, and (3) a layer of elastic fibers called **elastin.** The middle coat, or **tunica media,** is composed primarily of smooth muscle. The **tunica externa** or **adventitia** is the outermost layer or coat. It is composed principally of connective tissue. Although both veins and arteries have the same basic structure, arteries have relatively more muscle for their size than veins, and arteries appear rounder than veins because of this.

The blood pressure in the veins is insufficient to return blood to the heart, particularly from areas like the legs. Therefore, the flow of blood back to the heart is assisted by the massaging action on the veins of the skeletal muscles as they contract. This one-way flow of blood is ensured by the presence of *venous valves.*

Flow of Blood

The transportation of blood throughout the body is accomplished by the effort of two vascular systems: the arteries and the veins. Generally, veins have thinner walls than arteries and the blood in them is darker than that in arter-

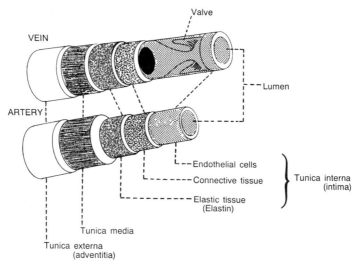

FIGURE 7.9 Comparative structures of a vein (top) and an artery (bottom). *AV,* atrioventricular; *SA,* sinoatrial.

ies because it is oxygen poor. Blood is carried *to* the heart through the **veins.** Blood flows **away** from the heart by way of the **arteries.** The following is an overview of the circulation of blood in the body. Actually, the process is much more complex, and it involves electric impulses plus a system of valves and muscle tone. Throughout the synopsis, please refer to Figure 7.10, which shows blood flow through arteries and veins.

1. Blood enters the upper right-hand chamber of the heart, which is called the **right atrium.**
2. Contraction occurs in the right atrium, and the blood passes downward into a second chamber called the **right ventricle.**
3. The right ventricle contracts, forcing the blood into a large blood vessel called the **pulmonary artery.**
4. The pulmonary artery carries the blood to the lungs where carbon dioxide is exchanged for fresh oxygen. Now the blood is oxygen-rich and bright red.
5. The blood flows from the lungs back to the heart through the **pulmonary veins.**
6. The pulmonary veins route the blood into the left upper chamber of the heart, which is called the **left atrium.**
7. Contraction of the left atrium pushes the blood into the most muscular chamber of the heart, the **left ventricle.**
8. Contraction of this chamber forces the blood into a large vessel called the **aorta.**

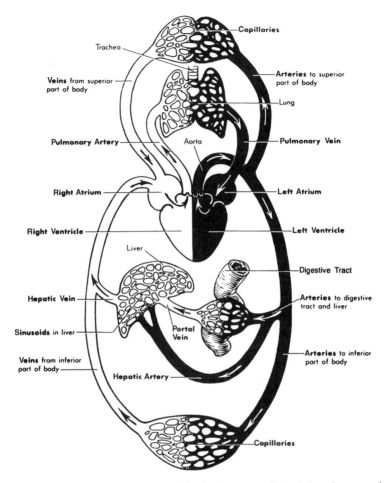

FIGURE 7.10 Schematic representation of the double system of circulation. Oxygenated blood is shown in black; the nonoxygenated blood is white. The arrows indicate the direction of flow. (Adapted with permission from Crouch JE. Functional human anatomy, 4th ed. Philadelphia, PA: Lea & Febiger, 1985.)

9. The aorta branches into subordinate arteries, which continue to divide and subdivide throughout the body until they become exceedingly small. The smallest arteries are called **arterioles.**

10. The arterioles subdivide into **capillaries,** which are thin-walled, microscopic pathways that connect with the veins.

11. Tissues give up carbon dioxide and waste products to the blood in the capillaries in exchange for oxygen and nutrients. This causes the blood to change from bright red to a darker hue.

12. The capillaries now lead into tiny veins called **venules.** The venules lead into progressively larger veins, which in turn lead into major **veins.**
13. The major veins now carry the blood to the two veins that return the blood to the right atrium of the heart—the **superior** and **inferior vena cava.** The cycle begins again.

BASIC COAGULATION

Coagulation is defined by Dorland's Medical Dictionary as " . . . the process of changing into a clot." Coagulation or clotting of blood is the action of three distinct components: (1) blood vessels, (2) blood platelets, and (3) coagulation factors. The collective action of the blood vessels and platelets in coagulation is known as primary hemostasis.

The blood vessels constitute the body's first line of defense. The vessels contract at the site of injury in response to various stimuli. This causes a decrease in blood flow and an aggregation of platelets.

Platelets are small cells that are normally found in the peripheral blood (Fig. 7.11). In addition to the role they play in coagulation, they also aid in the support of uninjured endothelial tissue. The platelets form a "plug" by adhering to the injured tissue. During this process, the platelets release their contents. These powerful contents are called aggregating agents, and they attract more platelets to the injured site. The aggregating agents also elicit further contraction of the blood vessels and are involved in the activation of the coagulation factors. A lack of platelet function or a decreased number of circulating platelets will affect the delicately balanced hemostatic scheme. As noted earlier, platelets are vital to the plug formation in vascular injury and in supplying phospholipids to the intrinsic pathway. The two primary tests for platelet activity are **bleeding time,** which is used to assess platelet function, and **platelet count,** which evaluates platelet production.

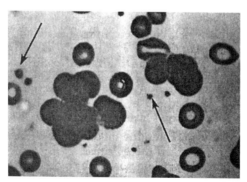

FIGURE 7.11   Photomicrograph of platelets. (Adapted with permission from Brown BA. Hematology: principles and procedures, 4th ed. Philadelphia, PA: Lea & Febiger, 1984.)

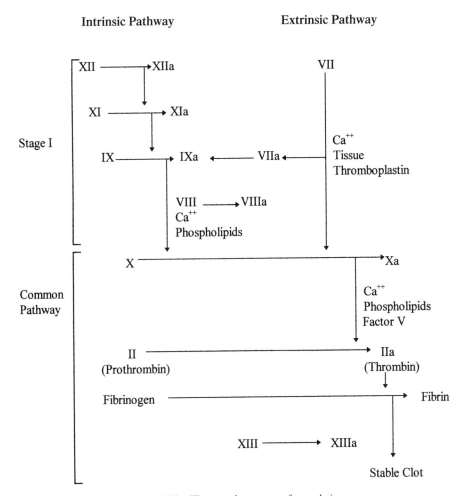

Intrinsic Pathway   **Extrinsic Pathway**

FIGURE 7.12   The cascade concept of coagulation.

The production of the fibrin clot, which requires coagulation factors, is known as secondary hemostasis. Secondary hemostasis has two pathways, the intrinsic and the extrinsic. These two pathways eventually join to form a common pathway, leading to the formation of a fibrin clot.

Each coagulation factor is assigned a Roman numeral, and the interaction of these factors has led to the "cascade" or "waterfall" concept (Fig. 7.12). The nomenclature for these coagulation factors has been established by the International Committee on Nomenclature of Blood Clotting Factors.

The activation of Factor XII initiates the intrinsic pathway. The system must go through a series of discrete activation steps before forming plasma thromboplastin. Factor XII converts Factor XI to the activated state. Now the activated Factor XI (XIa), in the presence of calcium ions and an activated Factor VII, enzymatically activate Factor IX (IXa). Activated Factor IX appears to form a complex with Factor VIII (which it has activated), calcium ions, and phospholipids to activate Factor X. It is with Factor X that the common pathway begins.

The extrinsic pathway is activated when the blood (plasma) is exposed to a protein called tissue thromboplastin, which is released by injured tissue. The extrinsic pathway is able to bypass the discrete activation steps (known as stage I) in the intrinsic pathway because injured tissue supplies the thromboplastin directly to the system. In the extrinsic pathway, Factor VII, forming a complex with tissue thromboplastin and calcium ions, also activates Factor X.

From this point, the process is known as the "common pathway." Factor X, activated by both the Factor IX complex and the Factor VII complex, converts Factor II (prothrombin) into thrombin (IIa). Thrombin, in turn, cleaves the fibrinogen molecule. This alters the fibrinogen molecule so that it forms a fibrin clot, which is stabilized by Factor XIII.

Several tests are used to assess secondary hemostasis. The two most common ones are the activated partial thromboplastin time (APTT) and the prothrombin time (PT). The APTT is used to screen for deficiencies of clotting factors in the intrinsic pathway; the PT is used to evaluate the extrinsic pathway.

Once healing has occurred and the blood vessel has repaired itself, the clot must be removed. This is done by the fibrinolytic mechanism known as fibrinolysis. Plasma contains a substance known as plasminogen. Activation of the coagulation system results in the conversion of plasminogen into the protease plasmin. Plasmin removes the clot by breaking fibrin down into smaller and smaller fragments known as fibrin-split products. In addition to the removal of clots, the fibrinolytic system keeps the vascular network free of deposited fibrin or fibrin clots.

BIBLIOGRAPHY

Barber J. Basic coagulation. Laboratory Medicine 1978;9:40.

Bick RL. Clinical significance of fibrino (geno)-lytic degradation products (FDP) testing. Lab Lore 1981;9:681.

Boggs DR, Winkelstein A. White cell manual, 4th ed. Philadelphia, PA: FA Davis, 1983.

Brown BA. Hematology: principles and procedures, 5th ed. Philadelphia, PA: Lea & Febiger, 1988.

Diggs LW, Sturm D, Bell A. The morphology of human blood cells, 5th ed. Abbott Park, IL: Abbott Laboratories, 1985.

Finch CA. Red cell manual. Seattle, WA: University of Washington, 1969.

Graninick HR. Intravascular coagulation 1. Differential diagnosis and conditioning mechanisms. Postgrad Med 1977;62:68.

Hillman RS, Finch CA. Red cell manual, 5th ed. Philadelphia, PA: FA Davis, 1985.

Johns CS. Hemostatic abnormalities in cancer. Advance/Laboratory 1997;6(7):25.

McClatchey KD, ed: Clinical laboratory medicine. Baltimore, MD: Williams & Wilkins, 1994.

McKenzie SB. Textbook of hematology. Philadelphia, PA: Lea & Febiger, 1988.

Steinberg D. Disseminated intravascular coagulation. American Journal of Medical Technology 1973;39:392.

Tortora GJ, Anagnostakos NP. Principles of anatomy and physiology, 6th ed. New York: Harper and Row Publishers, 1990.

The Blood Collection System

COLLECTION SYSTEMS

A variety of systems are now on the market that may be used to obtain and collect blood samples for clinical testing. The basic types are the evacuated blood collection system, the nonevacuated blood collection system, or syringe, the blood lancet, and the butterfly needle device.

Evacuated Blood Collection System

This system, which is the most widely used system for collecting blood samples (Fig. 8.1), consists of a collection needle, a holder, and an evacuated glass or plastic tube containing a premeasured vacuum. Sterile needles used with the evacuated system are packaged in plastic cases (Fig. 8.2) and are available in different lengths (e.g., 1 inch, 1½ inches) and gauges (e.g., 20, 21, 22). The shields are color-coded for quick gauge identification.

Nonevacuated Blood Collection System—Syringe

This system, although not used as extensively as the evacuated blood collection system, remains an important system for the collection of blood samples. It is primarily used for the collection of blood cultures and on individuals whose veins are difficult to stick. Like the evacuated blood collection system, this system is entirely disposable. As noted in Figure 8.3, the syringe consists of a barrel (which is graduated into milliliters) and a plunger. Needles may either be already attached to the syringe or packaged similar to needles used with evacuated blood collection systems. Needles used for one system are not compatible with the other.

1. Sterile needle. -

2. Rubber sleeve, making this needle suitable for multiple draws.

3. Holder that is used to secure the needle during insertion into the tube stopper during a venipuncture. - - - - - - - - - - - - - -

4. Evacuated glass or plastic tube. The tube comes in different sizes and the "stoppers" are color-coded to denote type of additive or no additive. - - - - - - - - - - - - - - - - -

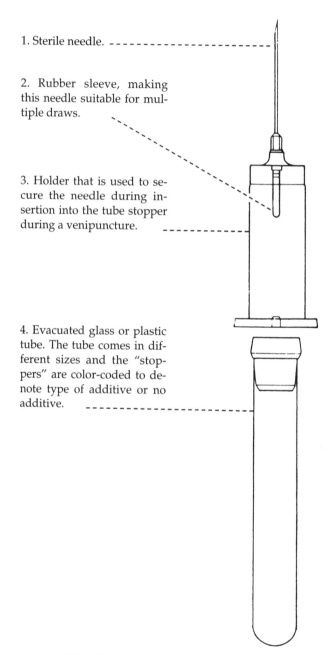

FIGURE **8.1**   Evacuated blood collection system.

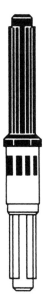

FIGURE 8.2 Coded plastic case containing sterile needle.

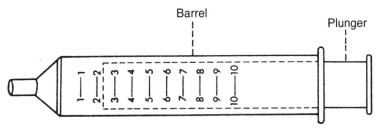

FIGURE 8.3 Syringe. (Adapted with permission from Brown BA. Hematology: principles and procedures. 4th ed. Philadelphia, PA: Lea & Febiger, 1984.)

Blood Lancets

The blood lancet is used for the collection of blood specimens by skin puncture. The lancet shown in Figure 8.4 is all metal and is available in individually sealed sterile packages. The tips come in different lengths. Several modifications are available. They are usually spring-loaded and have puncture depth control. These will be discussed in more detail in Chapter 10.

The Butterfly Needle Device

It was stated earlier that the syringe is useful in the collection of blood when the patient has veins that are difficult to stick. The butterfly collection device (Fig. 8.5) is becoming more popular. It is particularly useful on very young

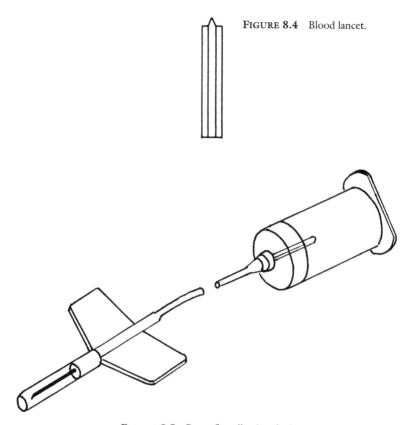

FIGURE 8.4   Blood lancet.

FIGURE 8.5   Butterfly collection device.

children and adults with extremely fragile and small veins. The "wings" allow the fingers of the phlebotomist to be closer to the needle so there is greater control and easier positioning when performing a challenging venipuncture. The butterfly used for blood collection has a flexible tubing attached with a needle or luer adapter on the opposite end. This allows for blood collection using either an evacuated blood collection device or a syringe. The butterfly needles are available in either 21, 23, or 25 gauge.

HOW THE PRIMARY ANTICOAGULANTS WORK—THEIR ADVANTAGES AND DISADVANTAGES

An anticoagulant prevents the blood from clotting by removing or neutralizing one of the essential factors necessary for coagulation. The anticoagulants routinely used in the clinical laboratory either (1) precipitate calcium, (2) bind calcium, or (3) inhibit thrombin.

Precipitate Calcium

Ammonium, lithium, potassium, or sodium oxalate prevents the coagulation of blood by removing calcium ions by precipitation as insoluble calcium oxalate. Using potassium oxalate as an example, the general or empiric formula is as follows:

$$K_2C_2O_4 \cdot H_2O + Ca \rightarrow CaC_2O_4 + K^{++}$$

A mixture of ammonium and potassium oxalate (double oxalate) is available primarily for use in Wintrobe sedimentation rates. Also, sodium oxalate is sometimes used in coagulation studies. However, the oxalates cause crenation of the red blood cells and bizarre forms of lymphocytes and monocytes, making them unsatisfactory for routine hematology procedures.

Bind Calcium

Ethylenediaminetetraacetic acid (EDTA), sodium polyanethole sulfonate (SPS), and sodium citrate prevent coagulation by binding calcium. EDTA and SPS are chelating agents. Chelation involves the bonding of a metal (in this case calcium) to a molecule that has two or more polar groups (the amine and carboxy groups in EDTA as illustrated in the empiric formula below). When this happens, a complex molecule is formed, removing the availability of calcium for the coagulation process.

EDTA, which is also known as sequestrene and versene, is available as a free acid and as the di-, tri-, or tetra-salt. Potassium salt is recommended to be used in preference to the sodium salt because of its greater solubility. EDTA is used perhaps more than any other anticoagulant for hematologic procedures. SPS, which is a weak chelating agent, is primarily used in the collection of blood cultures.

Sodium citrate also binds calcium by forming a soluble complex. Its effect is easily reversible by the addition of calcium. Consequently, it is the anticoagulant of choice for coagulation studies. In addition, it appears to preserve

labile procoagulants. The general formula for the binding of calcium by sodium citrate is given below:

$$
\begin{array}{cc}
\text{H—O} & \text{H—O} \\
\mid \quad \parallel & \mid \quad \parallel \\
\text{H—C—C—O—Na} & \text{H—C—C} \\
\mid & \mid \qquad \diagdown \\
\text{O} & \text{O} \quad \text{O} \\
\parallel & \parallel \quad \diagdown \\
\text{HO—C—C—O—Na+Ca} \rightarrow & \text{HO—C—C—O—Ca} \\
\mid & \mid \qquad \diagup \\
\text{O} & \text{O} \quad \text{O} \\
\parallel & \parallel \quad \diagup \\
\text{H—C—C—O—Na} & \text{H—C—C} \\
\mid & \mid \\
\text{H} & \text{H}
\end{array}
$$

Inhibit Thrombin

Heparin is available as an ammonium, lithium, or sodium salt, and its action is thought to prevent the transformation of prothrombin to thrombin and thus not allow a fibrin clot to form. It is a good anticoagulant because it causes the least interference in clinical chemistry tests. Unfortunately, it is expensive. In addition, it is not recommended for the preparation of blood smears when using Wright's stain because it causes a blue background to form on the smear.

STOPPER COLOR CODING FOR THE MOST OFTEN USED EVACUATED SYSTEMS

Color	Characteristic	Additive	Minimum Volume of Blood for Accurate Results
Red Top	For collection of serum; in addition to routine chemistries, recommended for blood banking and therapeutic drug levels	None	Not affected
Red-Gray Top	For collection of serum; polymer gel; separates serum from cells when properly centrifuged; not recommended for blood banking or therapeutic drug levels	Clot activator and polymer gel	Not affected

STOPPER COLOR CODING FOR THE MOST OFTEN USED EVACUATED SYSTEMS (*continued*)

Color	Characteristic	Additive	Minimum Volume of Blood for Accurate Results
Lavender Top	For collection of whole blood hematology determinations	Liquid K_3EDTA and powdered Na_2EDTA	Full draw preferred but no less than 75% draw
Light Blue Top	For collection of whole blood for coagulation determinations	Sodium citrate	Full draw required
Gray Top	For glucose determinations; contains glycolytic inhibitor; may or may not contain anticoagulant	Glycolytic inhibitors sodium fluoride or lithium iodoacetate or combinations of sodium fluoride and anticoagulant potassium oxalate or lithium iodoacetate and anticoaglant lithium heparin	Not affected

STOPPER COLOR CODING FOR THE MOST OFTEN USED EVACUATED SYSTEMS (*continued*)

Color	Characteristic	Additive	Minimum Volume of Blood for Accurate Results
Royal Blue Top	For collection of plasma or serum for determinations (e.g.; trace element and nutrient studies and toxicology profiles) sodium heparin, Na_2EDTA, or none	For tubes with anticoaulants, full draw preferred but no less than 50% draw	
Yellow Top Tube	For collection of special determinations such as immunodeficiency panels or for collection of blood cultures	Acid-citrate-dextrose (ACD) solution for the preservation of red blood cells or sodium	Not affected
Green-Gray Top	For collection of plasma for chemistry determinations; polymer gel separates plasma from cells when properly centrifuged	Lithium heparin and polymer gel	Full draw preferred but no less than 75% draw
Green Top	For collection of plasma for chemistry determinations	Sodium heparin, lithium heparin, or ammonium heparin	Full draw preferred but no less than 3/4 draw

STOPPER COLOR CODING FOR THE MOST OFTEN USED EVACUATED SYSTEMS (*continued*)

Color	Characteristic	Additive	Minimum Volume of Blood for Accurate Results
Brown Top Tube	For collection of plasma for blood lead determinations	Sodium heparin	Full draw preferred but no less than 75% draw

NOTE: Color coding given for both evacuated tubes with rubber stoppers and evacuated tubes with plastic closures.
EDTA, ethylenediaminetetraacetic acid.

PROBLEM SOLVING

General Problems	Possible Causes	Action
1. Short draw	Missed or transfixed vein Incomplete filling of tube	Redraw specimen if vein cannot be located. Allow tube to draw specified amount, thereby exhausting the vacuum. Check vacuum by filling another tube with water. Use tubes before expiration date.
2. Tube breakage during centrifugation	Unbalanced centrifuge	Balance centrifuge before use by using shields matched by weight.
3. Hemolyzed specimen	Traumatized specimen	Redraw specimen with a trauma-free venipuncture.
4. Poor (mushy) clot formation or poor clot retraction	Insufficient clotting time	Allow specimen to clot completely.
5. Presence of fibrin strands in serum tubes	Insufficient clotting time	Allow specimen to clot completely before centrifugation.

PROBLEM SOLVING (*continued*)

General Problems	*Possible Causes*	*Action*
6. Clotting in whole-blood (plasma) tubes	Insufficient mixing of additive with specimen	Mix well by inversion; make sure additive is not trapped around stopper by tapping tube lightly before filling.
7. Stopper pop-off during mixing of whole-blood tubes before repeat testing	Positive pressure created by reinserting stopper	Vent tube while reinserting stopper.
8. Incomplete barrier formation	Insufficient G force	Check centrifuge speed to make sure centrifuge is properly set to achieve force of 1200 G.
9. Peel-back of barrier	Use of angle-head centrifuge	Decant serum after centrifugation or use swing-head centrifuge.
EDTA		
10. False low hematocrit	Presence of excess EDTA owing to short draw	Check vacuum (see No. 1).
11. Cell distortion or hemolysis	Presence of excess EDTA caused by short draw or traumatic venipuncture	Check vacuum (see No. 1); redraw specimen with a trauma-free venipuncture.
12. False low white cell and platelet count	Clotted specimen	Mix specimen well by inversion (see No. 6).
Citrate and Oxalate		
13. Prolonged coagulation time	Short draw High hematocrit, as in polycythemia; the small amount of plasma in samples is inadequate to bind the available citrate	Check vacuum (see No. 1) to draw specified amount; use a reduced amount of anticoagulant.

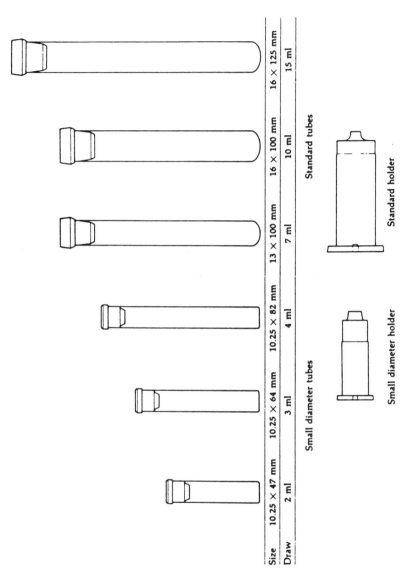

Size	10.25 × 47 mm	10.25 × 64 mm	10.25 × 82 mm	13 × 100 mm	16 × 100 mm	16 × 125 mm
Draw	2 ml	3 ml	4 ml	7 ml	10 ml	15 ml

Small diameter tubes   Standard tubes

Small diameter holder   Standard holder

FIGURE 8.6.   Commonly employed evacuated tubes.

PROBLEM SOLVING (*continued*)

General Problems	Possible Causes	Action
14. Low Westergren sedimentation rate	Incorrect ratio of citrate to specimen	Use tube with appropriate ratio of citrate to blood volume (1:4 recommended).
Heparin		
15. High sodium values	Sodium heparin salt interference	Use lithium heparin.
16. High lithium values	Lithium heparin salt interference	Use sodium heparin.
17. High BUN values	Ammonium heparin salt interference	Use lithium heparin.

BUN; blood urea nitrogen; EDTA; ethylenediaminetetraacetic acid.

TUBE AND HOLDER SIZE

Figure 8.6 illustrates the most commonly employed evacuated tubes and the proper size of holder to use with the tubes. The amount of blood that is supposed to be drawn is provided with each tube.

BIBLIOGRAPHY

1. A guide to the VACUTAINER brand evacuated blood collection system. Rutherford, NJ: Becton Dickinson Co., 1976.
2. Blood collection: monoject. St. Louis, MO: Sherwood Medical, 1990.
3. Brown BA: Hematology: principles and procedures. 5th ed. Philadelphia, PA: Lea & Febiger, 1988.
4. Focus on safety: a guide to Safety-Lok, Microtainer, and Vacutainer Tubes. Franklin Lakes, NJ: Becton Dickinson, 1993.
5. Henry RJ, Cannon DC, Winkelman JW, eds. Clinical chemistry: principles and techniques. 2nd ed. New York: Harper & Row, 1974.
6. Wiseman JD. Evacuated tubes and additives for blood specimen collection. 4th ed. Wayne, PA: National Committee for Clinical Laboratory Standards, 1996.

Procedure for a Routine Venipuncture

A patient's veins are the main source of blood for laboratory testing and a point of entry for IVs and blood transfusions. Because only a few veins are easily accessible to laboratory and other medical personnel, it is important that everything be done to preserve the vein's good condition and availability.

EQUIPMENT

1. Tourniquet
2. 70% alcohol preps
3. Sterile gauze pads
4. Evacuated tubes for ordered tests
5. Blood collection equipment (i.e., evacuated tube holder, syringe, butterfly needle)
6. Appropriate bandage

PROCEDURE

1. Review the request form(s). See what test(s) have been ordered, and confirm you have the appropriate blood collection equipment.

2. If the patient is confined to a health care institution, be sure to knock on the patient's door before entering the room.

3. Identify the patient. This is the *most important step* in the performance of a venipuncture.
   a. If the patient is conscious and competent, you may presumptively make an identification by asking the patient to verbally give their full name. This procedure should be followed on outpatients as well as inpatients.
   b. On inpatients, confirm the patient's identification by looking at the

wristband. Make sure that the name on the wristband and the name on the request form are identical.

   c. If the name on the request form does not match the name on the wristband or if no wrist band is present, have one of the nurses identify the patient. *Do not draw any blood until a positive identification has been made*. Note the nurse's name and the fact that the nurse identified the patient on the request form.

4. Let the patient know that you are from the laboratory and that you need to collect a blood sample for a test(s) that the patient's physician has ordered.

For patients that question the need for the venipuncture, emphasize that the patient's physician has ordered the test(s). This underscores its importance and necessity.

5. Check for required dietary restrictions.

If the test requires that the patient be fasting, make sure that these requirements have been followed. Also, if the patient is to have nothing by mouth (NPO [non per os]), you are not to give the patient anything to eat or drink, even if the patient asked for it.

6. Reassure the patient.

Gain the patient's confidence. Never say: "This won't hurt." Let the patient know that the venipuncture may be a little painful but will be of short duration. Many patients are reassured by polite conversation during the phlebotomy procedure.

7. Properly position the patient.

   a. If possible, have bed patients lie on their backs in a comfortable position. Do the same for any patient when you believe that the prone position would be safer for them or would make it easier for you to perform phlebotomy. Add support under the arm with a pillow if needed. Extend the arm so as to form a straight line from the shoulder to the wrist.

   b. Ambulatory patients or outpatients should be comfortably seated in a venipuncture chair. The arm should be positioned on an armrest in a straight line from the shoulder to the wrist. The arm should not be bent at the elbow.

   c. Make sure the patient does not have anything in his or her mouth.

   d. *Never* do a venipuncture on a patient who is standing.

8. Select and prepare your equipment (i.e., blood collection tube[s], needle holder, gauze, alcohol prep, etc.) before you apply the tourniquet. Wash hands, and make sure you have put on the appropriate personal protective equipment.

   a. Check the requisition form again for tube verification.

b. Select the proper size needle. The choice of needle usually depends on the size of the vein. The most frequently used needle is the 21 gauge. The gauge number indicates the diameter of the needle. The higher the gauge, the smaller the diameter. The length of the needle (1 to 1½ inches) is the choice of the phlebotomist.

c. The collection tray and assembled venipuncture equipment should be placed on a stand next to the patient, *not* on the patient's bed or person.

9. **Select site for venipuncture.**

Application of Tourniquet (Figs. 9.1–9.4)

Wrap the tourniquet around the arm approximately 3 to 4 inches above the area where you are going to "feel' for a vein (Fig. 9.1). Hold one end taut (Fig. 9.2). Then tuck a portion of the end under the taut end so as

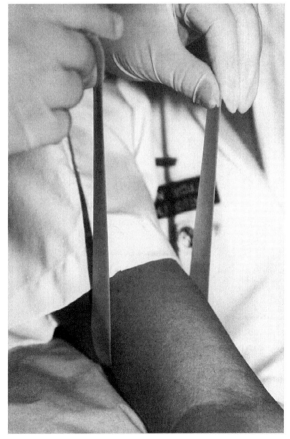

FIGURE 9.1 Wrap the tourniquet around the arm approximately 3 to 4 inches above the area where you are going to "feel" for a vein.

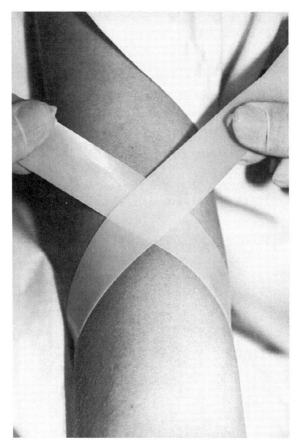

FIGURE 9.2   Hold one end taut as shown here.

to form a loop (Fig. 9.3). If applied correctly, the tourniquet should look similar to that in Figure 9.4.

Vein Selection

a. The three veins primarily used for venipunctures are the cephalic, basilic, and median cubital (Fig. 9.5).

b. Have the patient make a fist (this usually make the veins more prominent); however, vigorous pumping should be avoided. In some cases, it may be helpful to apply a warm damp washcloth to the area for 3 to 5 minutes so that the veins will become more prominent. However, do so with extreme caution. What may be warm to you, may be hot to the patient.

c. Using the index finger, palpate (feel) for a vein. Even if you can see the vein, palpate across the vein so you can be certain of its location and direction. A vein feels much like an elastic tube and "gives" under

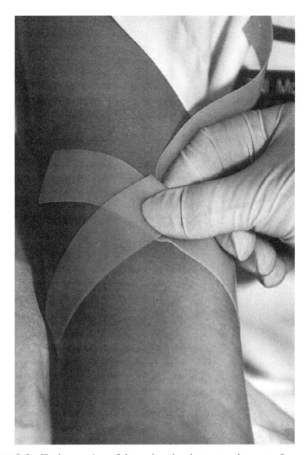

FIGURE 9.3   Tuck a portion of the end under the taut end so as to form a loop.

pressure. Also, veins do not pulsate as arteries do. If you have difficulty finding a vein, examine the other arm if possible. Sometimes veins in one arm will be more prominent than in the other. Take your time, find the best vein, but never leave the tourniquet on for longer than *one to two* minutes.

    d. Release the tourniquet before you clean the venipuncture site.

10. Clean the venipuncture site.

    a. Remove the alcohol prep from its package.

    b. Cleanse the vein site with a circular motion from the center to the periphery.

    c. Allow the area to dry. You may fan the area with your hand, but do not blow on the site.

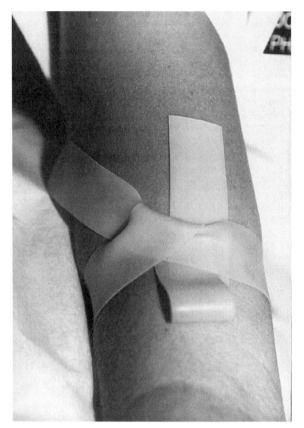

FIGURE 9.4 Front view of tourniquet on arm. To release the tourniquet, carefully pull the end of the tourniquet on the left.

    d. If the venipuncture is a difficult one and you have to palpate for the vein after you have cleansed the site, repeat the cleaning procedure.

11. Reapply the tourniquet.

12. Grasp the patient's arm approximately 1 to 2 inches below the venipuncture site. Pull the skin tight with your thumb to keep the vein from rolling.

13. Perform the venipuncture.
    a. If an evacuated tube is used, insert the tube into the holder and onto the needle up to the recessed guideline. Do not push pass this line because it will cause a loss of vacuum.
    b. The needle should be at approximately a 15 to 30 degree angle to the patient's arm and in a direct line with the vein (Fig. 9.6).

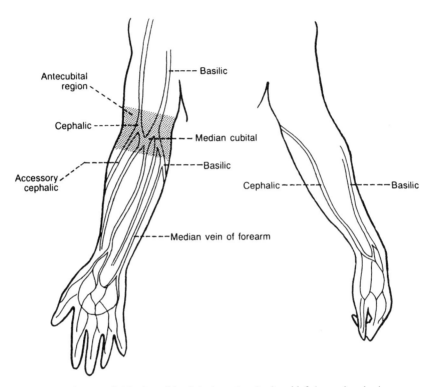

Antecubital region

Basilic

Cephalic

Median cubital

Basilic

Accessory cephalic

Cephalic

Basilic

Median vein of forearm

FIGURE 9.5 Superficial veins of the right (anterior view) and left (posterior view) arms.

c. The syringe or tube should be below the venipuncture site to prevent backflow, and the arm should be placed in a downward or level position.

d. Turn the needle so that the bevel is in an upward position.

e. Make the insertion in one swift motion until you feel the needle positioned in the lumen of the vein. Take care that the bevel of the needle is not against the vein wall thus obstructing blood flow or has penetrated the vein, which could cause a hematoma.

f. If a syringe is used, care must be taken not to pull on the plunger too rapidly or forcefully.

g. If an evacuated tube is used, as soon as the needle is in the lumen of the vein, while holding the needle holder firmly, use the free hand to push the tube as far as it will go. Steady the needle holder so that the needle is not inadvertently removed from the vein, causing a "short draw."

h. If multiple samples are drawn, continuing to keep the needle holder steady, carefully remove the active tube as soon as the blood flow stops and insert the next tube into the holder.

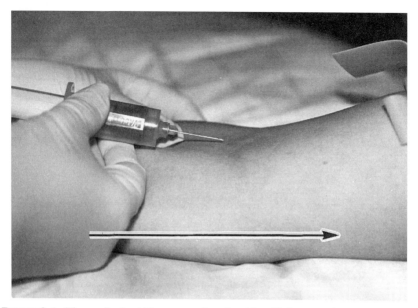

FIGURE 9.6   The needle should be at approximately a 15 to 30 degree angle to the patient's arm and in a direct line with the vein.

    i. Those evacuated blood collection tubes with additives should be inverted as recommended by the manufacturer. This should be done immediately and gently.

    j. Using a butterfly needle for phlebotomy:

        1) Carefully choose a suitable vein for phlebotomy.

        2) Clean the site as previously described.

        3) Palpate the vein noting the degree of vein stability.

        4) Assemble the necessary butterfly equipment. Butterfly needles have lines attached that can either lead to a head that screws into a syringe or to a needle suitable for insertion into evacuated tubes. Syringes should be used when veins are fragile or thin; evacuated tubes can be used when larger amounts of blood are needed.

        5) Perform the phlebotomy by inserting the butterfly needle carefully into the vein. Butterfly needles work best by lowering the insertion angle so that it is parallel to the hand and following the position of the vein (Fig. 9.7). After noting blood flow into the attached line, either pull back gently using the attached syringe or introduce the attached needle into an evacuated tube.

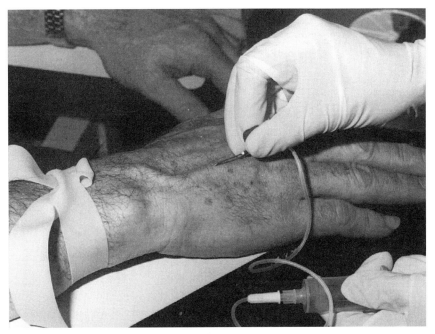

FIGURE 9.7   Hand phlebotomy using a butterfly needle. Note the lowered angle of the butterfly needle parallel to the hand.

14. Release the tourniquet.
The tourniquet may be release as soon as blood enters the tube or syringe or you may leave the tourniquet in place during the entire procedure.

15. If the patient continued to hold a fist during the procedure, now have them open their hand.

16. Place a square of sterile gauze over the puncture site, and quickly remove the needle (Fig. 9.8).

17. Apply pressure until the bleeding has stopped, then place a plastic adhesive pressure strip over the venipuncture site.
Some patients are allergic to plastic adhesive pressure strips. In these cases you may wish to cover the site with a hypoallergenic paper tape.

18. Label tubes.
Each institution has its own requirements regarding the labeling of specimen samples, however, the minimum should include: the patient's name, time the specimen was collected, date the specimen was collected, and the initials of the collector.

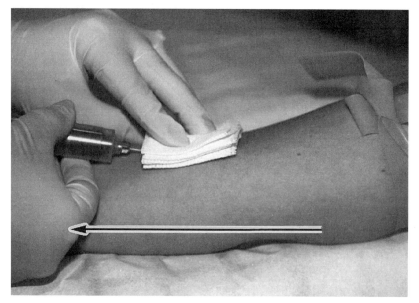

FIGURE 9.8 Place a square of the sterield gauze over the puncture site and quickly remove the needle.

19. *Properly* dispose of needles; remove and dispose of gloves; wash hands.

20. If in a patient's room, make sure to remove all equipment, making certain to collect and properly dispose of all contaminated equipment. Inpatient or outpatient—be sure to THANK them.

QUALITY ASSURANCE

1. Do not stick above an intravenous infusion (IV). If an IV is running in both arms and no other vein is available except in the area of the IV administration, specimens may be drawn *below* the IV site as follows: a) With the attending physician's permission, have the nursing staff turn off the IV for no less than 2 minutes before attempting the venipuncture. b) Apply the tourniquet *below* the IV site. A vein other than the one with the IV should be used. c) After performing the venipuncture, withdraw 5 ml of blood. *Discard.* Then draw the blood sample that is to be tested.

2. If you notice the venipuncture area beginning to swell while you are drawing blood, *immediately* release the tourniquet and remove the needle. Apply firm pressure on the venipuncture site for 7 to 10 minutes using several gauze squares. If possible, elevate the patient's arm while ap-

plying pressure. You may also wish later to apply an ice pack to the area. Watch the patient closely for any signs of fainting, vomiting, or other problems.

3. Do not keep the tourniquet on a patient's arm more than 1 to 2 minutes. Prolonged tourniquet application can cause significantly increased cholesterol, iron, lipid, total protein, and AST levels.

4. Outpatients should be seated for approximately 15 minutes before a venipuncture is attempted. Exercise and stress may cause elevations in the lactate dehydrogenase (LDH), AST, platelet count, and creatine kinase (CK) levels.

5. Make sure that all tubes have the appropriate draw. Refer to Chapter 8 for the minimum requirements. The National Committee for Clinical Laboratory Standards (NCCLS) recommends that health care facilities may wish to evaluate samples of their evacuated tubes to determine if they meet the labeled draw requirements under standard test conditions. The procedure is as outlined as follows:

   a) Fill a buret with deionized water.
   b) Bleed the connecting tube and needle to remove air.
   c) Refill the buret, and bring the meniscus to "0".
   d) Insert the needle attached to the connecting tubing into but not through the stopper of the evacuated tube.
   e) Open the stopcock of the buret, push the needle through the stopper, and allow the tube to draw until it stops.
   f) Read the volume of water drawn to the 0.1 ml after elevating the tube so that the meniscus in the evacuated tube is at the same height as the meniscus in the buret.
   g) Close the stopcock, and record the volume drawn.
   h) Each evacuated tube not falling within ±10% of the labeled draw should be deemed defective.

      Example: Let's say that a tube labeled as a 5 ml draw is evaluated. This means that 5.0 ml of deionized water should be withdrawn from the buret ± 0.5 ml. In other words, if the buret showed that no greater than 5.5 ml or no less than 4.5 ml of deionized water had been withdrawn, it could be reasonably assumed that the lot number of evacuated tubes was not defective.

6. Randomly selected samples of evacuated tubes should also be tested to determine if the stoppers function properly during collection and mixing. The following procedure is recommended by the NCCLS:

   a) Properly attach a 20-gauge non-lubricated blood-collecting needle to a syringe filled with deionized water.
   b) Push the needle through the stopper of an evacuated blood collection tube.
   c) Allow the tube to fill.

d) Slowly withdraw the tube, and observe the stopper to assure that it does not pull out of the tube.

e) Clean the stopper face of any residual water.

f) Without tightening the stopper if it has partially loosened, place the tube in a mechanical tube-mixing device and allow the device to operate for 20 minutes.

h) At the completion of the mixing, examine the stopper assembly for the following defects: stopper looseness and leakage of water in needle puncture point or around stopper.

i) The evacuated tubes shall be determined defective if the stopper pulls out, falls out, there is gross looseness, or any evidence of leakage.

7. The order of tube draw is possibly one of the most important considerations when performing a venipuncture using the evacuated blood collection system. This is because there is a risk of contaminating a subsequent tube with the additive from a tube just collected. For example, if a tube containing the potassium salt of ethylenediaminetetraacetic acid (EDTA) is collected prior to a tube for electrolyte evaluation, it is possible that the potassium value could be falsely increased. Likewise, the order in which

Evacuated Tube System

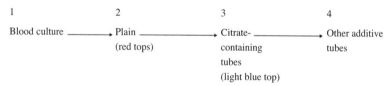

If several different additive tubes are to be filled, then the extended order of draw is as follows:

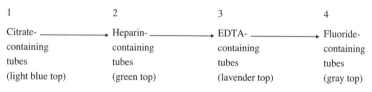

Syringe System

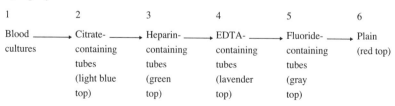

FIGURE 9.9. A suggested order of draw.

blood is added to tubes when a syringe is used is important because of the possibility of micro clots, which can cause erroneous coagulation and hematologic results. The recommended order of draw is outlined in Figure 9.9. Still under discussion is whether or not red top tubes containing a gel separator or thrombin should be treated as additive tubes.

BIBLIOGRAPHY

1. Brown BA. Hematology: principles and procedures. 5th Ed. Philadelphia, PA: Lea & Febiger, 1988.
2. DaCunha JP, Ford RD, Glover SM, eds. Diagnostics. Springfield, PA: Intermed. Communications, 1981.
3. Faber VL. QA/QC key to obtaining quality specimens. Advance 1997;9(15):6.
4. Garza D, Becan-McBride K, eds. Phlebotomy handbook. 4th ed. Stamford, CT: Appleton and Lange, 1996.
5. Kiechle FL. So you're going to collect a blood specimen. 6th ed. Northfield, IL: College of American Pathologists, 1996.
6. Maxwell R, Maxwell H, Parker CR, et al. Phlebotomy: The learning laboratorian series. Augusta, GA: Medical College of Georgia, 1989.
7. National Committee for Clinical Laboratory Standards: Procedures for the handling and processing of blood specimens. Approved Guideline H18–A. Villanova, PA: NCCLS, 1990.
8. National Committee for Clinical Laboratory Standards: Procedures for the Collection of diagnostic blood specimens by venipuncture. 3rd ed. Approved Standard H3–A3. Villanova, PA: NCCLS, 1991.
9. National Committee for Clinical Laboratory Standards: Evacuated tubes for blood specimen collection. 3rd ed. Approved Standard H1–A3. Villanova, PA: NCCLS, 1991.
10. National Committee for Clinical Laboratory Standards: Evacuated tubes and additives for blood specimen collection. 4th ed. Approved Standard H1–A4. Villanova, PA: NCCLS, 1996. *Permission to adapt portions of H1–A4 (Evacutated tubes and additives for blood specimen collection. 4th ed.; Approved Standard) has been granted by NCCLS. The complete current standard may be obtained from NCCLS, 940 West Valley Road, Suite 1400, Wayne, PA 19087 U.S.A.*
11. Statland BE, Boke H, Winkel P. Factors contributing to intra-individual variations of serum constituents: 4. Effects of posture and tourniquet application on variation of serum constituents in healthy subjects. Clin Chem 1974;20:1513.

Procedure for Skin Puncture

Skin or capillary punctures may be used to collect blood on patients of all ages; however, the skin puncture technique is primarily used on adult patients on whom it is difficult to perform a venipuncture or on whom the testing procedure requires capillary blood. Meites and Levitt gave two main reasons for collecting blood by skin puncture on infants: (1) micro volumes of blood are desirable to avoid anemia and (2) if needed, veins must be reserved for parenteral therapy.

EQUIPMENT AND SUPPLIES NEEDED

1. 70% alcohol preps
2. Dry sterile gauze
3. Appropriate size lancet
4. Collection containers suitable for specimen

PROCEDURE

1. Select the puncture site.

2. If necessary, warm the puncture site to increase the flow of blood.

   *When performing finger sticks on adults, this is not as much a necessity as when performing heel sticks on infants. In adults, holding the patient's hands between your hands and gently massaging the finger will usually suffice. Infant heels may also be warmed in this fashion or wrap the area for approximately 3 minutes in a moist towel with a temperature that **does not exceed 44 degrees Celsius.***

3. Clean the puncture site similarly to the procedure used when performing a venipuncture. After application of the alcohol, make sure the area is completely dry by wiping with a sterile gauze.

4. When performing a heel stick on an infant, hold the heel gently but firmly. This may be done in one of two ways: (1) place the forefinger around the ankle and the thumb over the arch of the foot (Fig. 10.1) or (2) place the forefinger over the arch of the foot and the thumb below the puncture site at the ankle. Use only lancets with a maximum length of 2.4 mm. Make the puncture perpendicular to the puncture site. Punctures should be made on the most medial or most lateral portion of the plantar surface (shaded areas in the diagram of an infant's foot (Fig. 10.2). Do not perform skin punctures on the posterior curvature of the heel.

   The depth of the skin puncture in the heel is important in infants, particularly neonates. It must not exceed 2.4 mm. Penetration of the calcaneous bone, osteomyelitis, and sepsis have all been reported as potential complications.

5. For a finger stick, place your thumb above and well away from the puncture site. The procedure is similar to that for the heel. The stick should be made into the pulp of the finger (as shown in the shaded area in Figure 10.3). The puncture should not be directed toward the bone. This will usually require a 10 to 20 degree angle to the longitudinal axis of the phalangeal bone.

   If a disposable lancet is used, such as the one illustrated in Figure 8.4 in Chapter 8, remember, the pain of a deep puncture is no more than that for a superficial one. You get a better flow of blood, and you may spare the patient from having to be stuck again.

6. Wipe away the first drop of blood using a dry gauze. (This is because the first drop may be contaminated with tissue fluids.)

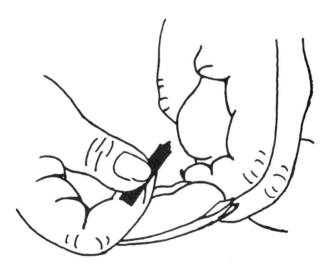

FIGURE 10.1 Proper positioning for heel stick.

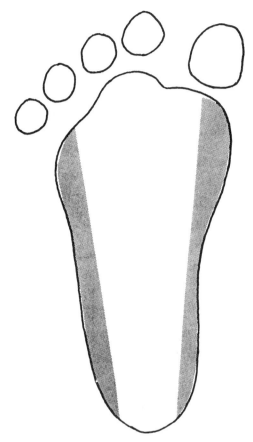

FIGURE 10.2   Diagram showing the areas (shaded) of an infant's foot that may be used for skin puncture.

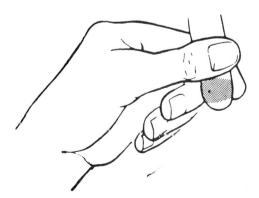

FIGURE 10.3   Area of fingertip puncture (Adapted with permission from Brown BA: Hematology: principles and procedures. 4th ed. Philadelphia, PA: Lea & Febiger, 1984).

7. Moderate pressure may be applied, but do not tightly squeeze or vigorously massage the area.

8. Collect the blood in an appropriate container.

9. Label with pertinent information such as patient's name, time and date of collection, and the collector's initials.

SKIN PUNCTURE DEVICES

In addition to the disposable blood lancet illustrated in Figure 8.4 in Chapter 8, an assortment of spring-loaded puncture devices are currently available on the market. Three examples are illustrated in Figures 10.4 through 10.6. Most spring-loaded puncture devices are available with lancets of varying depths and widths. Some spring-loaded puncture devices are totally disposable, others use only disposable lancets with the spring-loaded portion being

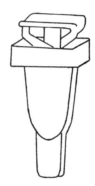

FIGURE 10.4   Safety flow lancet.

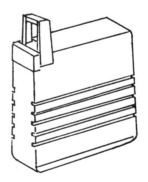

FIGURE 10.5   Tenderfoot lancet.

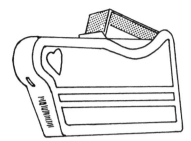

FIGURE 10.6   Tenderlett lancet.

reusable. The primary aim of these spring-loaded devices is to keep skin damage to an absolute minimum and to make obtaining a capillary puncture less painful, faster, and, in certain situations, hopefully a little less frightening.

Research is now being performed on the use of laser skin perforation for the collection of capillary blood. This technology presumably opens a hole in the skin by vaporizing the water molecules. It is anticipated that the use of this type of technology will improve patient comfort by reducing pain and lingering soreness, not to mention the reduction of medical waste by eliminating the need for skin lancets.

CAPILLARY BLOOD COLLECTION SYSTEMS

A number of micro collection systems currently available on the market have greatly simplified the collection and transportation of blood obtained from skin punctures. Three examples are illustrated (Figs. 10.7 through 10.9). Micro collection systems are available with or without an anticoagulant. Micro collection systems are also available with a separator gel for serum collection.

QUALITY CONTROL

1. Be sure to always use appropriate personal protective equipment.
2. Do not stick a baby's heel more than twice to obtain a blood sample.
3. Make sure the area for the skin puncture is completely dry before carrying out the procedure.
4. Be certain of the proper length lancet for the type of capillary puncture to be performed.
5. Remember not to squeeze the finger or heel too tightly so as to avoid diluting the blood with tissue juices or causing a bruise.
6. Collect the anticoagulated blood samples first to avoid microclots, then collect the specimens that require serum. Be sure to invert the anticoagulated tubes several times to prevent clotting.
7. After the capillary puncture is completed, apply gentle but firm pressure to the site until the bleeding has stopped. If necessary, an adhesive pres-

FIGURE 10.7   Microtainer with FloTop
Collector.

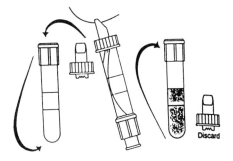

FIGURE 10.8   StatSampler.

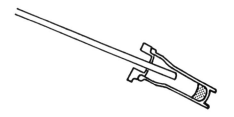

FIGURE 10.9   Sarstedt 1 ml capillary
blood collection system.

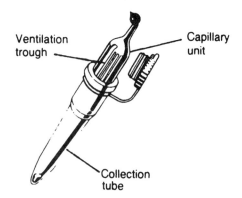

sure bandage may be applied to adults, but *never* use an adhesive pressure bandage on infants or neonates.

8. Be sure to note on the request form that the specimen was taken from a capillary puncture.

9. Make sure to properly label all specimens.

BIBLIOGRAPHY

1. Cell Robotics International, Inc. Lasette. Available at http://www.cellrobotics.com/cell/LASETTE.html. Accessed August 14, 1997.

2. Meites S, Levitt MJ. Skin-puncture and blood-collecting techniques for infants. Clin Chem 1979;25;183.

3. Phelan S. Blood collection: the pediatric patient. Chicago, IL: ASCP Press, 1990.

4. Randolph VS. Considerations for the clinical laboratory serving the pediatric patient. American Journal for Medical Technology 1982;48:7.

5. Simson E. Procedures for the collection of diagnostic blood specimens by skin puncture. 3rd ed. Approved Standard H4-A3. Villanova, PA: NCCLS, 1991.

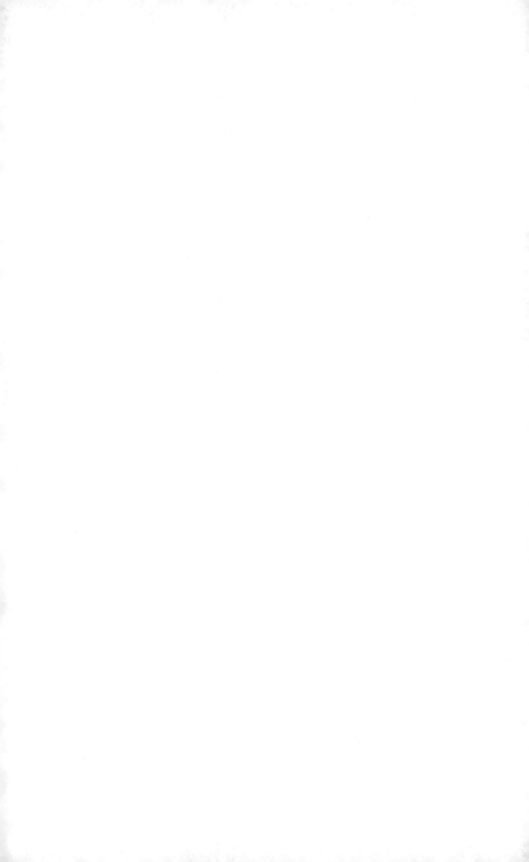

Special Situations in Phlebotomy

Fortunately, the majority of blood collections performed are "routine." But when confronted with special situations or problems, it is important that the phlebotomist act in a knowledgeable and professional manner. This chapter covers general guidelines for several of the more common situations or problems that may occur. Refer to Chapter 9 for what to do if a hematoma forms and instructions for the collection of blood from patients with intravenous infusions. *It is very important that each phlebotomist be familiar with and strictly follow the established guidelines at their own healthcare facility.*

PATIENT REFUSES TO ALLOW VENIPUNCTURE

If an adult patient refuses to be stuck, attempt gentle persuasion by reminding the patient that their physician needs the results of the laboratory tests to aid in the patient's treatment. *Never argue or get upset with the patient (or with the patient's family), and never touch the patient without their consent or subject them to any form of duress.*

Report this problem to the nursing station if you are in a hospital situation. Often patients will respond to reasoning by nurses when they will not listen to or cooperate with anyone else. If the patient still refuses, report the patient would not allow a blood collection to the appropriate supervisor. Request the nurses to notify the attending physician of the situation. Document the refusal on the laboratory request. When an adolescent refuses a venipuncture, the same procedure should be followed as for an adult—even if the parents give their permission for blood collection and offer their support.

If a child refuses to be stuck, the parents should be consulted. If the parents are willing and give their permission to attempt the blood collection, their assistance in securing the child is not only physically supportive, but also gives physical evidence of their consent. If the parents do not offer their assistance or give their permission, the appropriate individuals must be notified and the refusal noted on the laboratory request.

It is important to remember that when a child needs medical attention, particularly if admitted to the hospital, the parents may be distraught and even suffer from an unwarranted sense of guilt. Consequently, the parents might react belligerently toward anyone whom they perceive as inflicting additional and unnecessary pain on their child. It is important to be sensitive to their feelings and always be as tactful as possible.

DIFFICULT VENIPUNCTURE

Unfortunately, not all veins are prominent and easy to stick. From time to time, even good phlebotomists have difficulty in obtaining blood. It can be important to listen to the patient. Patients who have their blood drawn frequently know and will tell you which arm has the best vein(s) or if the veins are difficult to stick. You may make the decision that it would be better to have someone more experienced or who has stuck the patient previously to perform the venipuncture. If after palpating for a suitable vein, you decide to attempt a venipuncture, and if for some reason you cannot get any blood, try only once more. If, after the second attempt, you still did not get a specimen, notify the nursing station and/or the appropriate laboratory supervisor of the problem. This is particularly important if it is a timed specimen (e.g., glucose tolerance).

It was noted in a previous chapter that if the veins in one arm do not appear suitable for venipuncture, the other arm should be examined. If it appears, however, that drawing blood from the veins in either arm would be difficult, other sites should be examined and considered. These include veins in the hands, legs, and feet. *A word of caution:* venipunctures performed on the hands, feet, and legs are both difficult and potentially dangerous. The phlebotomist attempting to obtain blood from these sites must be knowledgeable regarding the proper technique. The veins of the hands are small, thin-walled, and have a tendency to roll, which makes them difficult to stick. Also, an abundant supply of nerves is located in the hands. This not only makes venipunctures in the hands more uncomfortable for the patient, but may cause potential complications because of nerve damage. Venipunctures in the legs and feet are most often performed on the elderly. This group of patients frequently suffers from varicosity, which results in venous stagnation; thus, venipuncture sites in these areas heal slowly. Both the hands and feet are notoriously contaminated with bacteria. This greatly increases the chances of infection from any invasive technique.

PATIENTS WITH MASTECTOMY

If at all possible, do not take blood specimens from the arm on the side of a mastectomy. If lymph nodes were removed, this will make the arm on the side of the mastectomy more susceptible to infection. Also, the laboratory results from blood taken on the side of the mastectomy may not be accurate because of possible lymphostasis. If a venipuncture must be done on that arm, use utmost precaution. Note on the requisition that blood was obtained from the arm on the side of a mastectomy.

THE FAINTING PATIENT

Fainting most often occurs because the patient is overly concerned about having blood taken. Fainting or syncope is the result of blood leaving the head, hands, and feet and collecting in the trunk of the body. There are several warning signs that a patient might faint. These include: 1) restlessness, 2) sweating more than usual, 3) paleness, and 4) deep breathing that is usually accompanied with sighs.

If any of the symptoms occurs while collecting blood, continue with caution. However, if several of the symptoms occur, it is best to discontinue the phlebotomy procedure. Have the patient lower their head to their knees. After the patient feels stable, move the person to a flat, comfortable surface such as an examination table or nurses' couch and have them lie down while you perform the phlebotomy procedure.

If the patient does faint (lose consciousness), lower the head immediately. Call for assistance and quickly and gently lower the patient to the floor. Clear the area of all obstructions, and closely observe the patient in order to make sure that no injury occurs.

Let the patient lie on the floor until recovered, then move them to the examination table or nurses' couch. Have the patient lie there for at least 15 to 20 minutes before allowing them to get up. Check the patient closely before they leave the phlebotomy area. If the patient is alone, do not let them drive. Seek assistance from family or friends, or get the patient a taxi. It is important to be reassuring to the patient because they may be embarrassed that they fainted. Let the patient know that fainting is common, and advise the patient to request in the future to have their blood drawn in a prone position.

Occasionally fainting patients may have symptoms similar to a grand mal seizure such as jerking, thrashing movements, and even urinary incontinence. This should not be mistaken as such, but do keep in mind that anxiety may trigger seizures in individuals with epilepsy. Upon recovery, a tingling sensation in the hands and feet may be experienced. Let the patient know that these will disappear. *In a fainting situation if the patient does not respond appropriately, seek emergency medical assistance immediately!*

VOMITING

If a patient begins to vomit during blood collection, immediately stop the procedure and control any bleeding. Call for assistance in supporting the patient to prevent the likelihood of fainting or aspiration. If possible, obtain some type of collection vessel such as a trash can. Using a cool wet towel, wipe the perspiration and vomitus from the individual's face. Remain calm, show understanding; always act in a professional manner.

THE PATIENT WITH AN IMPAIRED MOBILITY

Patients with Parkinson's disease or patients who have restricted physical movement (e.g., arthritis or limb abnormalities) present special problems in blood collection. Each situation is unique. Regardless of the situation, it is important that the phlebotomist act in a professional manner. Be gentle, sympathetic, and friendly, but not condescending. If necessary, do not hesitate to request assistance in steadying the area where the blood collection is to be performed.

BIBLIOGRAPHY

College of American Pathologists. So you're going to collect a blood specimen: an introduction to phlebotomy. 6th ed. Northfield, IL: College of American Pathologist, 1994.
Klosinski D. Blood collection: the difficult draw. Chicago, IL: ASCP Press, 1992.

SPECIAL TECHNIQUES

Special Collection Techniques

Most laboratory procedures in which blood is used require only a routine venipuncture. The sample must simply be collected in the correct tube. Several laboratory tests require distinctly special manipulations in addition to the venipuncture, such as prewarming the collection tube or administering a solution to the patient. Still other tests have nothing to do with venipunctures but are, nevertheless, invasive techniques that utilize one or more specific manipulations. This section does not attempt to discuss every laboratory test that requires special collection techniques; its scope is limited to those tests most often encountered.

PREPARATION OF A BLOOD SMEAR

Blood smears can be made from either capillary blood (finger/heel sticks) or venous blood. After the smear is prepared and air dried, the smear is usually stained with Wright's stain. Its primary use is for white blood cell differentiation and enumeration and morphologic studies. There are several different procedures for making blood smears, but the slide wedge method is the most commonly used.

THE SLIDE WEDGE PROCEDURE

1. 1×3 inch (25×75 mm) glass slides are used to make the slide wedge smear. The slides must be scrupulously clean. Questionably clean slides should first be soaked in 70% ethyl alcohol and then wiped dry with a lint free cloth.

2. A spreader must be used in the preparation of the slide wedge smear. Another 1×3 inch glass slide is most commonly used, and there are flexible plastic strips on the market, which may be used for this purpose.

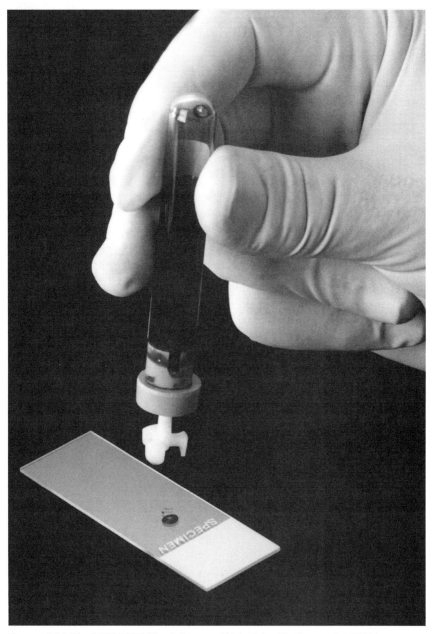

FIGURE 12.1 The DIFF-SAFE blood dispenser (Alpha Scientific Corporation [800] 242–5989).

3. If blood from a capillary stick is used, wipe away the first drop and use the second. Venous blood may be applied directly from the syringe or evacuated system needle. If a smear must be made later after the needle assembly has been removed, a device is currently available that has a cannula that may be inserted through the rubber stopper of the evacuated tube. The dispensers are either pressed against the slide (Fig. 12.1) or the blood is allowed to flow onto the slide (Fig. 12.2). The dispensers are designed to release an ideal drop size for making smears and eliminate the need to remove the stopper from the blood tube.

4. Regardless of the method of delivery, the drop of blood should be no more than 1 to 2 mm in diameter. Place the drop in the middle of the slide toward the frosted end. It should be approximately 1 cm in front of the

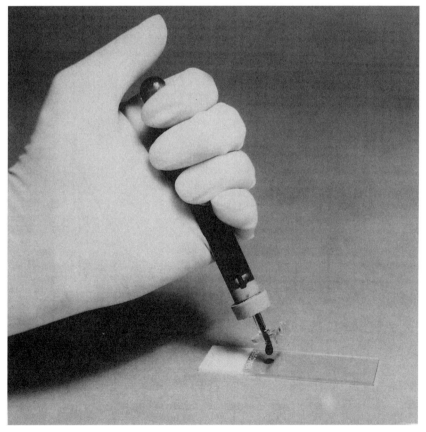

FIGURE 12.2 The H-Pette uses heat transfer from hand to tube to allow a drop of blood to flow through the cannula onto the slide. An attached blade may be used to make the smear. (Reprinted with permission from Helene Laboratories [800] 231–5663.)

frosted portion. Make the smear immediately after you have applied the drop of blood.

5. Place the slide on a flat surface, and hold securely. Use the thumb and index finger of the other hand to hold the spreader.

6. Place the end of the spreader just in front of the drop of blood at an angle of 25° to 30° (Fig. 12.3). Two main conditions affect the viscosity of blood: polycythemia (hemoglobin of 18 g/dL or greater) will increase the viscosity of the blood, and anemia (hemoglobin of 7 g/dL or less) will cause a decrease in the viscosity. When the viscosity is increased, a thinner slide is needed. To accomplish this, decrease the angle between the spreader and the slide. When the viscosity is abnormally low, a thicker slide is in order. To make thicker slides, increase the angle between the spreader and the slides.

7. Now draw the spreader back toward the drop of blood. Allow the blood to spread in the angle between the spreader and the slide. Just before the blood has spread to the edges, push the spreader ahead of the drop of blood.

8. Push the spreader the entire length of the slide. Make sure that you hold the spreader firmly against the other slide and that you make the smear in one smooth movement. Avoid any jerky movements.

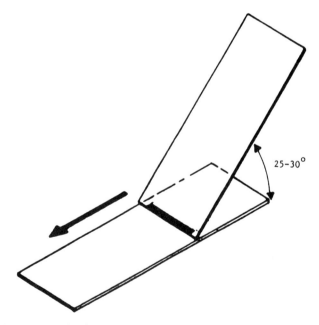

25–30°

FIGURE 12.3 Proper angle of spreader when preparing a slide wedge smear. (Adapted with permission from Bauer J. Clinical laboratory methods. 9th ed. St. Louis, MO: CV Mosby, 1982.)

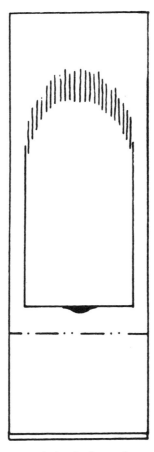

FIGURE 12.4 Diagrammatic sketch of properly prepared blood smear.

9. Air dry in a horizontal position. The smears are now ready for staining. A well-prepared blood smear has a thick portion beginning at the point of application that is drawn out into a feathery edge (Fig. 12.4).

BLOOD CULTURE COLLECTION

Because of the high risk of mortality caused by septicemia, it is imperative that the collection of blood for culture be performed as correctly as possible. Also, there are increasing occurrences of "normal flora" causing true infections, which make it critical that blood cultures are not inadvertently contaminated. Each health care institution uses its own particular blood culture system and has its own protocol for the collection of blood cultures. Nevertheless, certain procedural steps are common to all blood culture methods.

1. Examine the broth in the blood culture bottle before taking the blood sample. Discard if there is any evidence of contamination.
2. After removing any protective cap on the blood culture bottle, if present, disinfect the exposed rubber stopper.
3. Select a vein as you would for any other venipuncture.
4. Using a 70% alcohol swab, vigorously clean the area where the venipuncture is to be made, making concentric rings from the inside out. Let air dry. Do not touch the site. If the vein must be palpated again, do so only after the gloved finger of the collector is disinfected in an identical fashion as the arm. In addition to the 70% alcohol, a 2% tincture of iodine or povidone-iodine may also be applied before collecting the blood culture. Povidone-iodin is applied in a similar fashion as the alcohol, and it is allowed to dry before attempting the venipuncture.
5. The rubber stopper of the blood culture bottle should also be cleansed using either 70% alcohol or an iodine solution. Allow to set for 1 minute, then using a sterile gauze, remove any surplus disinfectant before injecting blood into the bottle.
6. Withdraw the blood using either a sterile needle and syringe or a closed system using a vacuum bottle. If a needle and syringe are used, inject the blood into the blood culture bottle. Do not change the needle before injecting the blood into the bottle. At least 10 ml of blood should be obtained each collection from adults. The physician should be consulted regarding the volume to be drawn from a young child. Usually 1 to 5 ml of blood each collection will be sufficient.
7. After the needle has been removed from the arm, apply pressure to the venipuncture site. If iodine was also used, again cleanse the site with 70% alcohol making sure that all iodine has been removed. Some patients are sensitive to iodine.
8. Gently but thoroughly mix the blood with the broth in the bottle. Properly label the blood culture bottle noting the patient's name, date, and time that the blood was drawn.

ORAL GLUCOSE TOLERANCE TEST

The purpose of the oral glucose tolerance test (GTT) is to confirm or aid in the diagnosis of patients with glucose metabolism disorders.

Preparation of Patient

1. The patient must not eat, smoke, drink coffee or alcohol, or exercise strenuously for at least 10 hours before or during the test.
2. If the GTT is to be performed on an outpatient, schedule the time the patient should arrive at the laboratory. Explain how many blood samples will

be required, and encourage the patient to bring something to read since the procedure will take some time to complete.

PHLEBOTOMY PROCEDURE

1. Obtain the patient's height and weight. Using these figures, calculate the amount of glucose solution to give the patient. A number of calculators are available to use for this purpose. An example of one such calculator is illustrated in Figure 12.5.

2. Draw a fasting sample. A fasting urine specimen may also be collected at the same time. Some institutions determine the glucose level of the fasting sample before administering the glucose solution. If the fasting glucose is high, the physician is contacted for instructions before the test is continued.

3. Give the patient the predetermined amount of glucose solution to drink. *Note the time.* Make sure the glucose solution is chilled. Instruct the patient to drink all the solution. This should be done within a 5-minute time limit. *Make sure you watch the patient drink the glucose solution.*

4. Draw a blood specimen at 30 minutes, 1 hour, 2 hours, and 3 hours (or more if required) after you have given the patient the glucose solution to drink. It may also be required that a urine specimen be collected after each time you stick the patient. Note the time each blood and urine sample was collected.

Special Considerations

1. The GTT is a timed test. Most patients on whom a GTT is being performed are borderline diabetics. As can be noted from the graph in Figure 12.6, in order for the physician to make a correct diagnosis, it is important that each specimen be drawn as close to the correct time as possible.

2. If, at any time during the test, the patient feels either faint or nauseated, have the patient lie down. It would be advisable to have an emesis basin and towel readily available just in case the patient needs to vomit. If vomiting occurs within the first half-hour of the test, discontinue, notify the physician, and if appropriate, reschedule for another day. On the other hand, if vomiting occurs approximately 1 hour and 15 minutes after the test has started, have the patient lie down, and complete the test. If, after repeated attempts to perform the oral GTT, the patient continues to vomit within the first half-hour, the intravenous (IV) GTT may have to be considered. If urine is collected during the testing period, encourage the patient to drink water to promote adequate urine excretion. If the patient

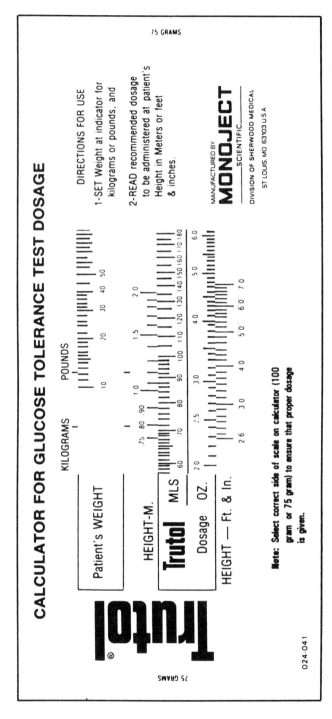

FIGURE 12.5 Example of a calculator used to determine the amount of glucose solution to be administered to a patient when performing the glucose tolerance test.

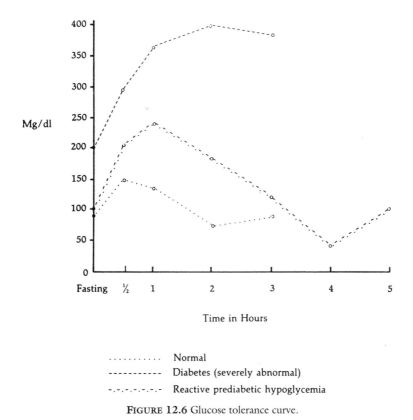

.... Normal

----------- Diabetes (severely abnormal)

-.-.-.-.-.- Reactive prediabetic hypoglycemia

FIGURE 12.6 Glucose tolerance curve.

should develop severe hypoglycemia, take a blood sample, note the time, alert a physician, and *discontinue the test.*

BLOOD SPECIMENS FOR CROSSMATCHES

When obtaining a blood sample from any patient, the greatest care must be exercised to make sure that the sample is taken from the correct patient and that the sample tubes are properly labeled. This statement cannot be made often and emphatically enough. *Nowhere is the above statement more important, however, than when obtaining a blood sample from a patient who may possibly need a blood transfusion.*

Ordering procedures vary but generally a *type and Rh* are ordered on all pregnant females. This may be known as a prenatal screen. The blood is typed to see whether it is type O, A, B, or AB and to see whether it is either Rh positive or Rh negative.

Surgeons will often order a type and screen on their patients scheduled for surgery who may need blood transfusions. This will be determined on the amount of blood loss during the operation. The type and screen include the type and Rh determinations and testing the patient's blood for the presence of specific antibodies. If the patient has an antibody and a transfusion is required during surgery, the blood bank will have had time to acquire compatible blood.

At present, blood is usually crossmatched before it is transfused. The word "usually" is used because there are situations, such as severe hemorrhaging, in which any blood is better than no blood and the time required for a cross-match makes it an impractical procedure.

The cross match basically includes the ABO type and Rh factor determinations, a screen of the recipient's blood for specific antibodies, and tests to see whether the recipient's serum has antibodies that will react against the donor's red blood cells—in other words, a check to see whether the donor's blood and the recipient's blood are compatible. Infusion of incompatible blood can cause clumping (agglutination) or rupturing (lysis) of the red blood cells in the recipient's circulatory system.

PHLEBOTOMY PROCEDURE

1. *Make sure of the patient's identity.* Do not ask "Are you Ms. Smith?" Ask the patient to state their full name. Next, check the patient's hospital identification arm band against the name on the requisition form. If the patient is unconscious or otherwise incoherent, *have a health care provider assigned to the area positively identify the patient.*

2. Draw at least one red top tube (*without polymer gel*), two if possible, and a purple top tube. Properly label the tubes.

3. Make sure to collect the blood specimens carefully so that hemolysis of the red blood cells does not occur.

4. Most hospitals have some type of identification band that is placed on the patient's wrist as soon as the specimen has been collected. The bands are usually made of soft plastic and must be cut to be removed after they have been attached.

5. There is also a label that has a preprinted identification number identical to the one on the wrist band. This label must be affixed to the tube of blood. This same identification number will be placed on the unit of blood that has been crossmatched. In addition to the patient's name and other information, the nurse, before infusing the blood, will check to see whether the identification number on the patient's wrist band corresponds exactly with the identification number on the unit of blood. *Remember, check and double check when obtaining a blood sample where there is a possibility that blood may be transfused.*

COLD AGGLUTININS

Everybody has cold agglutinins in their serum. They most strongly react around 4°C. Normal individuals have titers of less than 1:32 with titers of 1:256 or greater indicating a cold agglutinin disease. Cold agglutinin titers are most often used in supporting the diagnosis of *Mycoplasma pneumoniae*.

PHLEBOTOMY PROCEDURE

1. Collect the sample in a red-top tube. Approximately 30 minutes before sticking the patient, place the tube in a 37°C incubator to prewarm. In order to keep the tube as warm as possible, carry the tube in your palm when going to the patient's room.

2. After collecting the specimen, bring the tube back to the laboratory as soon as possible. Again, carry the tube in your palm. When you get to the laboratory, place the specimen into a 37°C incubator or water bath to clot. Alert testing personnel of the specimen. If the specimen is to be sent elsewhere for testing, separate the serum from the cells as soon as the specimen has clotted.

Special Considerations

Prevent hemolysis when collecting the sample. Also, if you allow the specimen to get cold, the cold agglutinins will coat the red blood cells and leave none in the serum for testing.

FIBRIN DEGRADATION PRODUCTS

From the basic coagulation scheme in Chapter 7, you will remember that thrombin induces clot formation by the conversion of fibrinogen to fibrin. If the process stopped there, all of us would eventually find our circulation impaired because we would be full of clots. But once a wound has healed, the clot is removed by the process of fibrinolysis. Plasmin digests fibrin (the clot), generating fibrin/fibrinogen degradation products (FDPs) called X, Y, D, and E. These degradation products have an anticoagulant action.

Sometimes a pathologic state occurs in which generalized clotting takes place in the small blood vessels. In fact, the clotting may be localized to one or a few organs. This phenomenon may be caused by infectious agents, solid-tumor malignancies, leukemia, or hemolytic disorders, to name just a few of the diseases. This complex entity is known as disseminated intravascular coagulation (DIC).

DIC is a paradox in that clotting occurs that causes bleeding. In other words, an excess of thrombin exists that causes enhanced clotting. The enhanced clotting stimulates excessive fibrinolysis (with its degradation products) and allows bleeding.

When DIC is suspected, the platelet count and fibrinogen determination (the two most important tests) are the minimum needed. The primary test for the confirmation of DIC involves detection of FDP.

PHLEBOTOMY PROCEDURE

1. Because DIC is a life-threatening condition, an early and accurate diagnosis is essential. Extreme care must be taken to avoid hemolysis of the specimens during collection.

2. Because a platelet count and fibrinogen level will be ordered, it will be necessary to collect specimens in both a purple top tube and a blue top tube. In addition, a red top tube specimen should be carefully collected so that possible hemolysis can be observed.

3. A commercial test is used in most laboratories to detect the presence of FDP. The specimen to be used for this test must be collected in a special tube containing thrombin and an antifibrinolytic agent. Mix gently after drawing.

BLEEDING TIME

The bleeding time, also known as the Ivy bleeding time, is an in vivo test for platelet and capillary function. Reference ranges vary somewhat according to the template used; therefore, the manufacturer's insert must be consulted. As a rule of thumb, 2 to 7 minutes is a normal bleeding time with variations attributed to gender and age. Regardless, concern is warranted for bleeding times greater than 12 to 15 minutes.

Preparation of the Patient

1. Explain to the patient that a bleeding time is a test to see how long it will take for the patient's blood to stop bleeding and to form a clot.
2. Unless circumstances indicate otherwise, outline to the patient how the test will be performed. Explain that the test will take approximately 10 to 20 minutes to complete.
3. Let the patient know that some discomfort may be experienced from the incision and the cuff of the sphygmomanometer.
4. Sometimes, the test is less traumatic and the time passes faster for children if their assistance is solicited in watching the stopwatch and letting the person performing the procedure know when to blot the blood.

PHLEBOTOMY PROCEDURE

1. The arm must be in a supine position on a steady support, with the volar surface exposed.

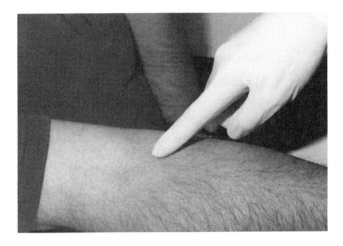

2. The incision is best performed 5 cm below and parallel to the antecubital crease. Avoid surface veins.

3. Clean the area with 70% alcohol. If the arm is very hairy, lightly shave the area.

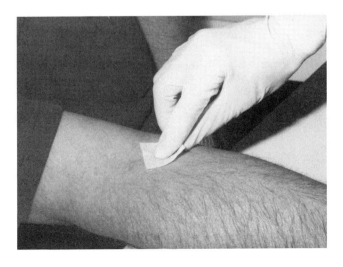

4. Remove the incision-making instrument from its package. Be careful not to contaminate the instrument by touching or resting the blade-slot end on any unsterile surface. Ready it for use by removing any safety devices.

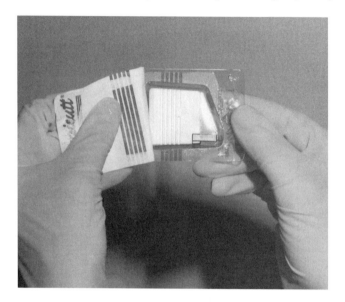

5. Place a sphygmomanometer cuff on the upper arm, and inflate to 40 mm Hg. Monitor the sphygmomanometer frequently to make sure the pressure remains at 40 mm Hg throughout the test.

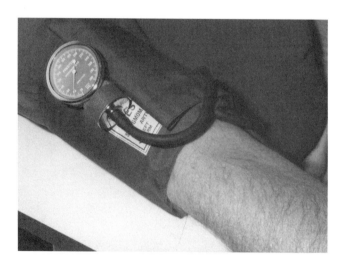

6. The test should be started within 60 seconds after the blood pressure cuff has been inflated. Place the incision-making instrument firmly on the forearm, but do not press. A horizontal incision is the most sensitive technique for the bleeding time test. Activate the trigger and start the stopwatch simultaneously. Remove the incision-making instrument almost immediately after activating the trigger.

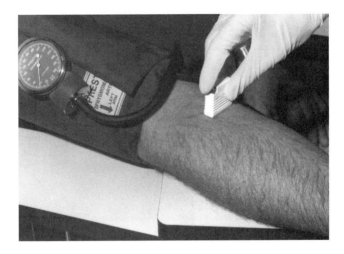

7. Blot the flow of blood every 30 seconds. Place the filter paper close to the incision, but do not touch the edge of the wound because this may disturb the platelet plug.

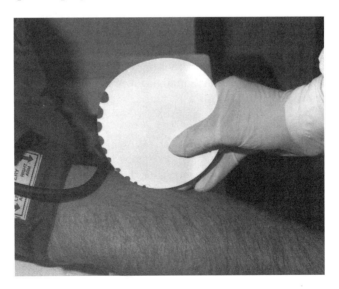

8. Continue to blot every 30 seconds until the blood no longer stains the filter paper. Stop the stopwatch, and note the time to the nearest 30 seconds.

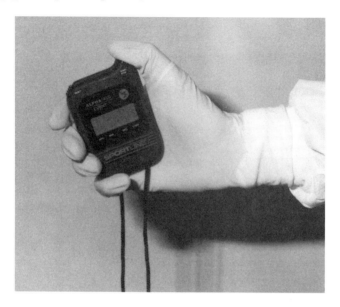

9. Remove the sphygmomanometer cuff. Gently clean the arm with an antiseptic swab, and place a butterfly bandage across the incision. The patient should keep the bandage in place for at least 24 hours.

Special Considerations

There are several situations when a bleeding time should not be performed. For example, when patients have edematous or excessively cold arms or low platelet counts or are taking medications containing aspirin. Bleeding times should also not be performed on individuals with sunburns and diseases of the skin.

ARTERIAL PUNCTURES

Arterial blood is used to evaluate gas exchange in the lungs by measuring the partial pressure of oxygen and carbon dioxide. *An arterial puncture is a dangerous procedure. Only those individuals who have been extensively trained in the technique should attempt to perform arterial punctures.* It is important when performing an arterial puncture that you be very honest with the patient. Explain what the procedure is and that it will be uncomfortable. Solicit the patient's cooperation, reminding the patient to remain still. However, *do not promise that cooperation will guarantee success.*

Pre-packaged kits are currently available that contain the necessary materials needed to perform an arterial stick. Most contain the following:

   a. A heparinized syringe with a 23-gauge needle attached
   b. A rubber stopper or cube
   c. Alcohol swab, gauze, and bandage

Depending on the length of time it takes to return to the testing area, a basin or zip-lock plastic bag containing crushed ice may be necessary. After preparing the materials needed to perform the stick, the following procedure should be followed:

1. Perform the Allen test to assess circulation. This is accomplished in the following manner:
   a. Rest the patient's arm on the bedside table, supporting the wrist with a rolled towel. Have the patient make a clenched fist.

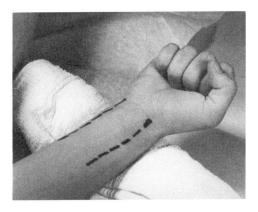

   b. Using the middle and index fingers of each hand, exert pressure on both the radial and ulnar arteries.

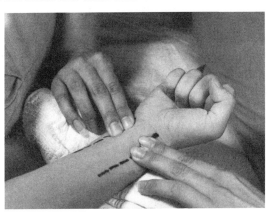

c. Without removing pressure, have the patient unclench the fist. Note the palm for blanching, which indicates impaired blood flow.

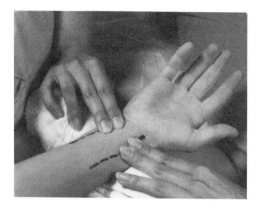

d. Release the pressure on the ulnar artery. Check to see whether the palm begins to turn pink in approximately 5 seconds. If it does not, this may indicate that there is possible occlusion of the radial artery or poor cardiac output. If this is the case, perform the Allen test on the other wrist.

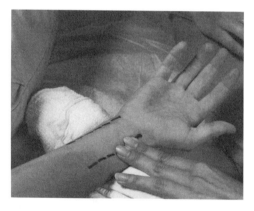

2. When trying to locate an artery, constant pressure with the middle and index fingers is the method of choice, rather than palpating, as is performed when trying to locate a vein. This is because the location of an artery must be performed by detecting a pulse.

3. Using a circular motion, clean the puncture site as you would for a venipuncture. Let the area air dry. In the same manner clean the gloved fingers that will be used to locate the artery.

4. While holding the syringe in one hand, use the free hand to once again make sure of the location of the artery.

5. Puncture the skin at a 45 to 60° angle. Advance the needle slowly. When you puncture an artery, the blood will "pulsate" into the syringe, pushing the plunger up of its own accord. *Avoid pulling back on the plunger if possible.* Carefully withdraw at least 1 ml of blood.

6. Never attempt to perform an arterial puncture more than twice, and *never probe.*

7. After you have obtained the sample, gently expel any air bubbles by holding the syringe in an upright position, and slowly force a small amount of blood out of the syringe into a gauze pad. Some collection devices are designed so that this problem does not occur.

8. Next stick the needle into the rubber stopper or cube to seal it from the air.

9. Mix the specimen gently but thoroughly.

10. It may be necessary to place the sample on ice for transportation to the laboratory.

11. After removing the needle, apply firm pressure to the puncture site for at least 5 minutes. After pressure is released, a bandage may be firmly taped over the puncture site. Do not, however, tape the entire wrist since this may restrict circulation. Never ask the patient to apply the pressure. The patient may not apply pressure sufficiently or for a long enough time.

12. After completing the procedure, properly remove gloves, and wash hands.

GENERAL PROCEDURE FOR THE UNOPETTE BRAND HEMATOLOGY SYSTEM

The UNOPETTE is a microcollection system developed by Becton Dickinson. It basically consists of a reservoir and a capillary pipette that is self-filling and self-measuring (Fig. 12.7). The system has been developed for manual use and for use with automated equipment. Individual UNOPETTE systems are available to perform a variety of hematology procedures such as white blood cell counts, red blood cell counts, platelet counts, eosinophil counts, and reticulocyte staining. Procedural variations exist between the systems, but the patient-sample collecting steps are basically similar, except for the reticulocyte determination. The UNOPETTE manual white blood cell count is described in the following section to illustrate the sample collection steps.

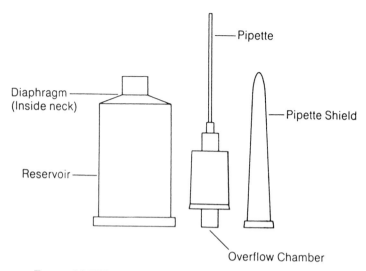

Pipette

Diaphragm
(Inside neck)

Pipette Shield

Reservoir

Overflow Chamber

FIGURE 12.7 The major components of the UNOPETTE system.

1. Place the reservoir on a flat surface, holding it securely with one hand. Using the other hand, firmly push the tip of the pipette shield through the diaphragm in the neck of the reservoir, and then remove the pipette shield.

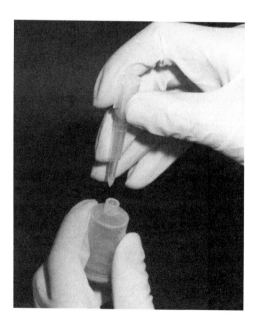

2. Next, remove the pipette shield from around the pipette by a simple twist.

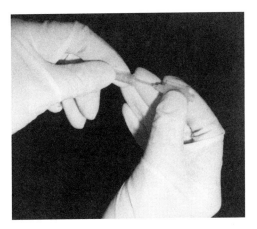

3. Hold the pipette almost horizontal while touching the tip of the pipette to the patient's blood. The pipette will fill by capillary action. The filling is complete and will stop automatically when the blood reaches the end of the capillary bore in the neck of the pipette.

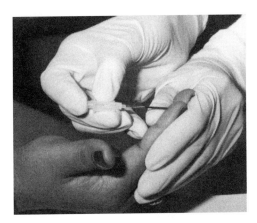

4. Wipe any excess blood from the outside of the capillary pipette, making sure that none of the sample has accidentally been removed from the bore of the pipette.

5. Next, squeeze the reservoir slightly to remove some of the air without expelling any of the liquid. Maintain this slight pressure on the reservoir.

6. Covering the overflow chamber of the pipette with the index finger, place the pipette securely into the neck of the reservoir.

7. Release the pressure on the reservoir, and remove the index finger from the pipette. The negative pressure will draw the blood into the diluent.

8. Squeeze the reservoir gently two to three times to rinse the capillary bore. Force the diluent up into, but not out of, the overflow chamber of the pipette. Release the pressure each time to return the mixture to the reservoir.

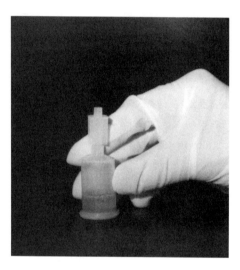

9. Now place the index finger over the upper opening (the inserted pipette), and gently invert the system several times to thoroughly mix the blood and the diluent.

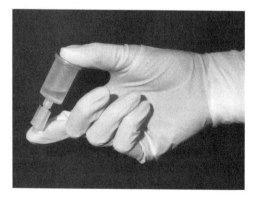

10. Convert to a dropper assembly by withdrawing the pipette from the reservoir and reseating it securely in the reverse position.

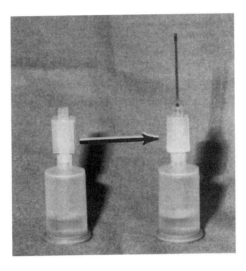

11. For transporting and temporary storage, place the capillary shield loosely over the exposed pipette.

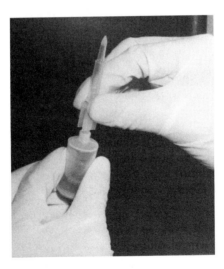

HEPARIN LOCK PROCEDURE

In rare situations, multiple draws must be made either in a short period of time (e.g., checking electrolytes) or as timed samples (e.g., the glucose or insulin tolerance test) on patients with veins that are next to impossible to locate, much less stick. This situation often occurs with debilitated patients (usually in the intensive and cardiac care units) or with extremely obese patients. In these situations, it may be appropriate to use a heparin lock. This allows the laboratory to obtain the required number of samples with minimum discomfort, not to speak of psychologic trauma, to the patient. Because heparin is a drug, the physician's permission will be required to insert this device. Also, this procedure is somewhat tedious and demands special precautions. Only approved individuals should attempt to insert and use the heparin lock.

Material Required

1. 21-gauge butterfly with heparin lock
2. heparin lock flush solution, 10 USP per ml
3. TUBEX hypodermic syringe
4. gauze
5. paper tape
6. tuberculin syringes
7. syringes with 21-gauge needles
8. IV support board

PHLEBOTOMY PROCEDURE

1. Surgically clean the area where the heparin lock is to be inserted.

2. Vent the heparin lock with a 21-gauge needle.

3. Insert the butterfly into the vein, and let the blood flow freely into the tubing and out the 21-gauge needle. Make sure that no air remains in the system.

4. Next, connect a syringe to the 21-gauge needle, and obtain the first blood sample.

5. Remove the syringe and the 21-gauge needle. Using a TUBEX hypodermic syringe, flush the heparin lock with 1 ml of the heparin solution.

6. Place the patient's arm on an IV support board, and secure the heparin lock using gauze and paper tape.

7. To obtain subsequent samples:
   a. Clean the surface of the heparin lock with 70% alcohol.
   b. Insert a tuberculin syringe with a 25-gauge needle, and slowly withdraw 1 ml of heparin-blood mixture. Properly discard.
   c. Quickly insert a 21-gauge needle attached to a syringe into the heparin lock. Slowly aspirate the desired amount of blood sample.

   d. Remove the needle and syringe. Place blood in appropriate evacuated tubes, and properly dispose of the needle and syringe. Again flush the heparin lock with 1 ml of the heparin solution as previously described.

   e. Repeat steps 7a through d, as necessary.

THERAPEUTIC DRUG MONITORING

Therapeutic drug monitoring is used to ascertain the probability of drug-induced disease and to determine any drug interactions and side effects. It is also used to monitor drug administration errors and patient noncompliance. The monitoring of all therapeutic drugs and all patients is neither feasible nor necessary. However when specimens are required for therapeutic drug levels, they must be drawn at specific times. These times are determined by how the drug was administered (i.e., oral or IV) and the drug's pharmacokinetics (e.g., half life of the drug, absorption rate). The physician may order **trough** and **peak** levels. A trough level is when the drug is at its lowest concentration in the blood. Usually this is just before the next dose is to be administered. The peak level usually occurs soon after a dose of the drug is administered and represents its highest concentration in the blood.

    When performing peak and trough levels on a patient taking a therapeutic drug, *communication* with the health professional administering the drug is vital. Proper timing in the collection of specimens is critical to determine the drug's concentration and establish its clinical effects. The trough level must be collected just *before* the next dose is given; while the peak level must be drawn exactly as possible at the same number of minutes *after* the last dose was administered.

NURSERY TECHNIQUES

Newborns and premature infants are at a high risk of infection because their immune systems are immature. Newborns become colonized with their mother's normal flora; however, newborns can pick up microorganisms from the personnel who work in the nursery. This can pose a potentially life-threatening situation. It is very important then that the phlebotomist be familiar with the proper procedures for nursery collections in the particular hospital in which they work. A general outline is given below:

1. If required, place disposable booties over shoes.
2. Wash hands as described in Chapter 6, and properly put on gloves.
3. Putting on a clean gown and disposable mask may be required. Under certain situations sterile gloves may also be required.
4. Take into the nursery *only those items needed to collect the blood specimen*.
5. After collection of the specimen, return to the anteroom to properly label.

6. If clean gown, mask, and booties were required, remove them at this time, and properly deposit them in approved receptacles. Wash hands.

BIBLIOGRAPHY

Bartlett RC, Ellner PD, Washington JA II. Blood cultures, Cumitech 1. Washington, DC: American Society for Microbiology, 1974.

Brown BA: Hematology: principles and procedures. 5th ed. Philadelphia, PA: Lea & Febiger, 1988.

Castle M: Hospital infection control, principles and practice. New York, NY: John Wiley and Sons, 1980.

DaCunha JP, Ford RD, Glover SM, eds. Diagnostics. Springfield, PA: Intermed Communications, Inc., 1981.

Gralnick HR. Intravascular coagulation. 1. Differential diagnosis and conditioning mechanisms. Postgrad Med 1977;62:68.

Johns CS. Hemostatic abnormalities in cancer. Advance 1997;6(7):25.

Kiechle FL. So you're going to collect a blood specimen. 6th ed. Northfield, IL: College of American Pathologists, 1994.

Laboratory procedure using the UNOPETTE brand system. Rutherford, NJ: Becton Dickinson, 1977.

McKenzie SB. Textbook of hematology. Philadelphia, PA: Lea & Febiger, 1988.

Reynolds JB. Detection of fibrinogen/fibrin degradation (split) products fdp/fsp. Research Park, NC: Burroughs Wellcome Co., 1981.

Patel K. Heparin lock procedure. Personal Communication, 1983.

Drawing Blood Donor Units

PREDONATION PROCEDURES

Welcoming Donors

It is important that donors be greeted and treated in a calm, professional manner throughout the donation process. This gives reassurance to first-time donors and those donors feeling nervous about the process of giving blood.

Checking Health History of Donor

Potential donors who are willing to donate blood must undergo a health history screening process to determine if their blood is healthy enough to be transfused to someone else. Potential donors first register by providing their name, social security number, date of birth, address, and telephone number. A donor may be asked to produce a picture ID to confirm the identity of the donor. Donors who are unable to provide an address or telephone number are discouraged from donating if they are unable to provide a reliable way to be contacted. A mini-checkup of vital signs, which consists of recording the donor's pulse, temperature, weight, and blood pressure, is performed on each donor to ensure their current health.

Nurses or other health care professionals screen applicants by personally interviewing each donor about their health and medication history. Questions about lifestyle are asked to eliminate the donors who are at risk of potentially spreading diseases transmissible through blood. The hemoglobin or hematocrit levels of the donor are taken to screen donors who may be anemic. Usually a single drop of blood from either a simple finger or ear stick is all that is needed. These values must fall within guidelines set by the blood bank or blood collection agency.

After donors have passed through the screening process and have been deemed acceptable to donate blood, they will receive a donor kit consisting

171

of an empty sterile blood collection bag with anticoagulant added that contains a small amount of clear colorless fluid. A sterile capped needle and one or more smaller empty bags, which are used to prepare blood components from blood in the main collection bag, are attached to the bag by long tubing. This set of connected bags is referred to as a "unit" (Fig. 13.1.). The numbering on the unit bag and the paperwork should match each other exactly and be unique. That is, no other donor should have the same number on their unit bag or donation paperwork.

Seating Donor on Phlebotomy Bed

To start the donation, the phlebotomist should welcome the donor, take the donor kit, and indicate where the donor should lie during the donation process. Donors should be asked to remove heavy sweaters or bulky coats. If a donor is wearing tight or restrictive sleeves, they should be asked to change into a provided smock. Donors may not chew gum or eat while on the donor bed because of the danger of accidental aspiration. Donors may donate from either the left or right arm, depending on their preference, but the phlebotomist makes a final choice based on vein suitability. Place the donor's purse or other possessions out of the way in a safe place, which is free from any possible contamination from an accidental blood spill. Some donors may be more comfortable if their legs and lap are shielded by a provided cover.

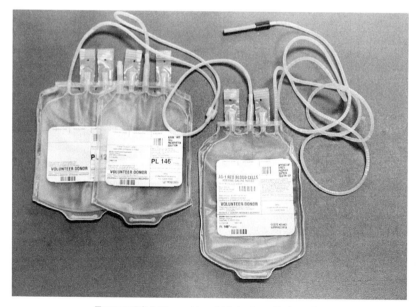

FIGURE 13.1 Donor kit, which is also called a unit.

At this point the phlebotomist is responsible for checking to make certain all the health history questions have been answered appropriately and that each vital sign falls within the stated guideline. The unique numbering of the paperwork and unit bag is checked to be sure they are identical. The phlebotomist then identifies the donors by asking them to verify data on their donation paperwork (e.g., confirm name, date of birth, and social security number). Any doubts about the suitability of the donor or any question about the paperwork should be resolved by a supervisor before proceeding with the donation process. The phlebotomist should then inspect the unit bag and tubing for any leaks, cracks, or discoloration while placing the unit bag on a scale in readiness for donation.

Vein Selection

The phlebotomist should inspect for the best donation site in the antecubital area of both arms. An appropriate donation site should be free from any skin punctures or scarring that is suggestive of self-injected drugs. The donation site should also be free of any skin disease or inflammation. If neither arm is acceptable, contact your supervisor.

Examine the donation site for a suitable vein by placing a blood pressure cuff or tourniquet of moderate tightness two inches above the antecubital space. While holding the pressure at 60 to 80 mm Hg or after the tourniquet has been fastened, have the donor squeeze a hand grip, and look for a distended vein large enough to hold a 16-gauge needle for the required time during donation. Usually the cephalic or median cubital veins in the center of the antecubital area are used. Using your finger, palpate the distended veins for elasticity, diameter, and tissue support. The basilic and accessory cephalic veins are located on the outside and inside of the antecubital area. These veins can be large enough to use for donation, but usually require more skill and care in the placement of the needle because of the "flattened" needle angle needed for a successful donation. After selecting the donation site, release pressure from the blood pressure cuff. Position the donor's arm exactly as it will be placed during phlebotomy; mark the position and base of the chosen veins that are not visible by pressing and slightly twisting the end of a cleaning swab into the skin at the phlebotomy site.

PHLEBOTOMY

Equipment Needed for Donation

Once a suitable vein is found, check to make certain that all supplies needed for the donation process are available. Supplies needed may include:

> Lap cover
>
> Blood pressure cuff or tourniquet

Hand grip

Paper or surgical tape

Benzidine iodine swabs

Alcohol-cleaning swabs

Clamps

Sterile gauze

Metal clamps and clamping device

Alcohol preps

Elastic bandaging

Blood line stripping device

Some equipment, such as a blood stripping device is specialized for blood donation (Fig. 13.2.). These items will be provided to the staff before beginning a donation.

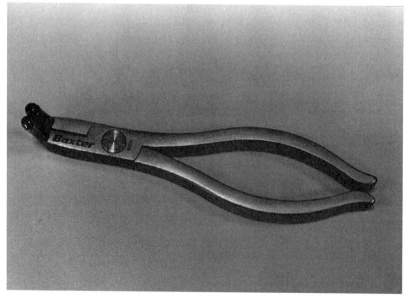

FIGURE 13.2 Blood stripping device.

Using Protective Equipment

Once a suitable vein is found and the necessary supplies have been gathered to draw a unit of blood, the phlebotomist should put on protective equipment. This consists of a lab coat or gown and gloves. The lab coat or gown should have long sleeves and cover most of the phlebotomist's clothing. The gloves should fit appropriately and can either be powdered or unpowdered. The gloves do not have to be sterile but should be changed between each donor. Gloves that are visibly contaminated need to be removed and replaced with clean gloves as soon as possible before proceeding, even if the donation has not finished. Although patient care is the first priority, all protective equipment should be changed at the first opportunity whenever it becomes visibly contaminated.

Gloves should be worn whenever there is a reasonable chance that hands will come in contact with blood or contaminated work surfaces. Some tasks that require wearing gloves include:

• Performing phlebotomies
• Handling filled blood unit bags
• Handling all blood specimen (stoppered and unstoppered) tubes
• Replacing bandages over phlebotomy sites
• Cleaning blood spills
• Cleaning equipment and work surfaces that are potentially contaminated

Cleansing the Donor Arm for Phlebotomy

1. Open a 7.5% povidone iodine solution; swab and vigorously cleanse an area at least two inches in every direction from the needle entry site. This should result in a 4-inch diameter circle of cleaned arm.
2. Open a 10% povidone iodine solution swab; starting at the center of the phlebotomy site, cleanse the arm in an outward spiral to the edge of the first iodine circle. Do not reclean any area after the second iodine is applied. The second iodine swab cleans the arm even more by pushing any remaining skin bacteria to the edge of the phlebotomy site.
3. Allow this area to air dry. Do not blow on this site to speed drying since this may introduce bacteria to the cleaned site.
4. If the phlebotomy is difficult and further palpation is required, repeat the cleaning procedure before attempting the venipuncture.
5. Donors who are allergic to betadine iodine may have their arms cleaned with two alcohol swabs in the manner described above.

Performing Phlebotomy

1. Before beginning phlebotomy, tape the line connected to the needle to the donor's arm with tape near the wrist of the arm chosen for donation.

Enough tubing should be left free from the taping to allow insertion of the needle in the antecubital area.

2. Make certain a clamp or hemostat is clamped onto the tubing between the needle and the taped tubing at the wrist before the needle is uncapped. This prevents air and possible contaminants from entering the blood bag after the needle is uncapped.

3. Reapply the blood pressure cuff to a pressure of 60 to 80 mm Hg or place a tourniquet of moderate tightness around the donation arm. Ask the donor to squeeze the hand grip, and tell the donor to expect venipuncture.

4. Stand in a direct line with the angle of the venipuncture, and uncap the needle. Inspect the needle for barbs or defects. If the needle is unsatisfactory, do not use it, and call for the supervisor.

5. Using the thumb of your free hand, pull back on the skin approximately 1 to 2 inches below the phlebotomy site to keep the vein from rolling. This action also lessens the pain of the venipuncture.

6. Hold the base of the needle with bevel up. At an angle of 30 to 40° and in line with the vein, penetrate skin smoothly without hesitation. The needle should be advanced $1/2$ inch into the lumen of the vein while conforming to the anatomy of the vein.

7. Relax the clamp on the needle tubing. If the venipuncture was successful, blood should immediately flow down the tubing toward the main unit bag. If no blood appears, slightly advancing the needle either into or out of the vein may be necessary to begin blood flow. Call your supervisor if neither of these actions result in blood flow. To probe any farther results in pain and agitation for the donor.

8. After blood flow begins, secure the needle hub to the donor's arm by placing a 4-inch piece of tape across the needle hub, attaching the needle to the donor's arm. Cover the venipuncture site with sterile gauze to maintain sterility of the area. This action also helps calm the donor by keeping the needle positioned in the donor's arm from their immediate view.

9. As blood begins flowing into the main unit bag, gently invert the bag to mix the anticoagulant and blood.

10. Check to see how the donor is feeling. Ask the donor to squeeze the hand grip every 5 to 10 seconds to aid the flow of donor blood into the unit bag. Invert the unit bag after every 100 ml of blood has entered to ensure mixing of the anticoagulant with the collected blood.

11. After the desired amount of blood has been collected, a hemostat clamp is replaced on the tubing between the needle and the tape holding the tubing near the wrist. (Hint: placing the clamp closer to the needle makes errant blood drops falling from the needle much less likely.)

12. Loosen the blood pressure cuff or tourniquet, and remove it from the donation arm.

13. The tape holding the donation tubing close to the wrist is carefully loosened. Be certain to avoid accidentally pulling the needle from the donor's arm after this step.

14. Next, place sterile gauze 2×2 squares over the needle tip resting in the vein and grasp the needle base with the other hand. Simultaneously remove the needle from the arm in one smooth motion and with the other hand press down firmly on the gauze over the venipuncture site to stem further bleeding.

15. Instruct the donor to raise their arm into the air while holding the gauze firmly over the venipuncture site for three to five minutes.

16. Push the needle into the vacutainer tubes attached to the main unit bag, and release the clamp to fill the tubes with blood. Make certain to clamp the tubing attached to the needle between filling each tube or air will enter the blood bag and contaminate the unit. The purple top tube is filled first, followed by the red top tubes. If one purple top and one red top tube cannot be completely filled with the donor's blood, perform a simple phlebotomy from the donor's other arm to fill the appropriate vacutainer tubes. A collected unit is useless without the minimum number of vacutainer tubes.

17. After the last tube has been filled, use the blood line stripping device to empty the blood content of the tubing into the main bag. With one hand, hold the end of the tubing firmly, while the other hand slides the tightly gripped stripping device along the tubing, emptying the contents of the tubing into the main blood bag (Figs. 13.3A and B. This permits blood in the tubing to become mixed with the anticoagulant in the main bag, which prevents clotting from occurring in the tubing. After releasing the stripping device from the tubing, blood will flow back into the tubing. This tubing is later sealed into portions to be used in the laboratory for crossmatching the unit of blood.

18. After the arm stops bleeding, clean the donor's arm by wiping the excess iodine from the arm using an alcohol prep. Be careful not to disturb the venipuncture site. Bandage the arm by placing a folded sterile 2×2 over the phlebotomy site, and secure this to the arm with a piece of tape or a stretch bandage.

19. Warmly thank the donors for their donation, and caution them against any heavy lifting activity with the donation arm for the next several hours. Encourage them to increase their fluid intake over the next several days. Release the donor for escort to the canteen area.

Recording Phlebotomy Information

To ensure quality, certain information about the donation must be recorded by the phlebotomist on the donation paperwork. Blood collection agencies

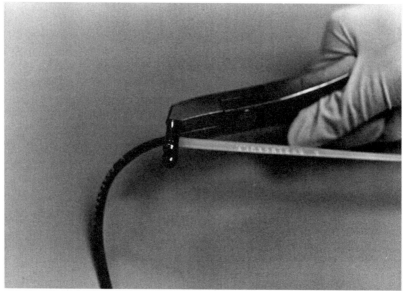

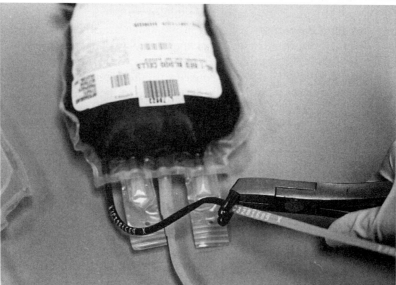

FIGURE 13.3 A and **B,** Tightly grip the stripping device along the tubing to empty the contents of the tubing into the main blood bag.

govern what specific information must be recorded. Generally, the time the donation was started and the arm used must be recorded.

Monitoring the Donation Process

The phlebotomist is responsible for care and support of the donor during the donation process. The rate of blood flow into the unit bag should be constantly monitored because the actions of a phlebotomist are necessary if complications such as bleeding problems or donor reactions occur. To avoid the risk of an air embolism, the base of the unit may be lifted to mix the anticoagulant with collected blood, but the unit bag should not be squeezed during donation. A supervisor should be consulted for patients with slow bleeds or when patients form hematomas.

Discontinuing Donation

Donations should be discontinued after the desired weight of donor blood is collected. Blood collection agencies collect 450 ± 45 ml of blood from adult donors. Too much blood or too little blood alters the anticoagulant:blood ratio to unacceptable levels for transfusion purposes. Therapeutic blood donations can be collected from donors weighing less than 110 lb. In this case, the amount of blood actually collected is decreased by 8 ml for every lb the patient weighs under 110 lb (4 ml of blood for every lb under 50 lb). The accurate weight of collected blood can be achieved by placing the main unit bag on a dietary scale set to 0 and allowing blood to fill the unit bag to the desired weight.

1. After the desired amount of blood has been collected, a hemostat clamp is placed on the tubing between the needle and the tape holding the tubing near the wrist. (Hint: placing the clamp closer to the needle makes errant blood drops much less likely.)
2. The blood pressure cuff or tourniquet is loosened and removed from the donor's arm.
3. The tape holding the donation tubing close to the wrist is carefully loosened. Be certain to avoid accidentally pulling the needle from the donor's arm after this step.
4. Next, hold 2×2 gauze squares over the needle tip resting in the vein and grasp the needle base with the other hand. Simultaneously remove the needle from the arm in one smooth motion and with the other hand press down firmly on the gauze over the venipuncture site to stem any further bleeding.
5. Instruct the donors to raise their arm into the air while firmly holding the venipuncture site covered by the gauze for 3 to 5 minutes.

6. Push the clamped donation needle into each vacutainer tube accompanying the unit bag, and release the clamp allowing the vacutainer tube to fill with blood. Make certain to reclamp the hemostat around the needle tubing between filling each tube or the needle will leak blood rather vigorously.

DONOR REACTIONS
Nervousness

It is the rare donor who does not admit to feeling some amount of nervousness before giving blood. For this reason, donors are comforted by a sense of professionalism in the donation area. Signs of nervousness may include the extreme quiet or overly boisterous behavior of donors before actual phlebotomy begins. Distracting the donor with general conversation often lessens their anxiety and leads to a pleasant donation experience for the donor.

Dizziness, Pallor, Nausea, and Fainting

Some, but by no means all, donors may experience discomfort during the donation process. Early intervention by a phlebotomist may interrupt these symptoms allowing for a successfully completed donation. At the first sign of symptoms in a donor reaction, the donor's feet should be elevated (approximately 25 to 30°) and head lowered (Fig. 13.4.). A cool cloth can be applied to the forehead if the donor complains of feeling warm. Slightly altering the position of the donor may be all that is needed to continue the donation process. However, the donation should be stopped by removing the needle if signs of discomfort continue or if the donor asks for the donation to stop.

For extremely nervous donors, a cool non-diet beverage can be offered to the donor once phlebotomy begins. (If the donor sips this beverage through a straw, there is much less chance of accidental aspiration.) Offering a beverage provides distraction that can calm a donor as well as meet the increased caloric needs of a nervous donor that are met by the sugar in a beverage.

Friends and relatives should not be allowed to group around a donor during a donation. Well-meaning individuals may agitate a donor and interfere with the phlebotomist's care if a donor reaction occurs.

Pain at the Phlebotomy Site

Phlebotomy at the donation site should not cause any undue pain after the needle's entry into the arm. Some donors may experience a stinging sensation in the area of venipuncture from the iodine or alcohol used for cleaning the arm. Continued pain at the phlebotomy site may call for a slight adjustment of the needle's placement in the donor vein. If the donor's pain cannot be resolved, the donation should be stopped to avoid any damage from occurring.

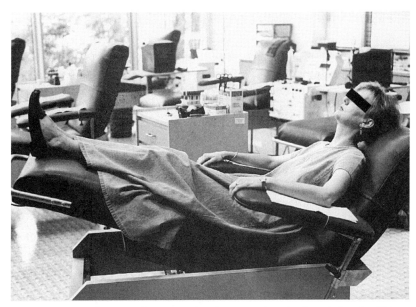

FIGURE 13.4 At the first sign of symptoms in a donor reaction, the donor's feet should be elevated approximately 25 to 30° and the donor's head should be lowered.

Some donors may experience a tingling sensation after the needle is removed. This symptom generally subsides after a few minutes. Lasting pain symptoms or the inability to move the donation hand freely should be investigated as soon as possible.

Hematoma

A hematoma may form at the site of phlebotomy. Some hematomas grow rapidly in size and are a sign that the donation should be stopped immediately because blood is escaping the vein and is entering tissue surrounding the vein. The donor should be advised that this area will bruise slightly, but fade as time passes. Any immediate pain and swelling can be controlled by giving an ice pack to the donor with instructions that it should be applied and removed at 10-minute intervals to the hematoma site for several hours after a donation.

POST-DONATION INSTRUCTIONS TO DONOR

Increased Fluid Intake

Donors should be advised to increase their fluid intake for 48 hours after their donation. Any symptoms they may experience after their donation will occur from the fluid loss that occurs as a result of donation, not from the actual loss of blood cells.

Reduced Heavy Lifting Activity

Any heavy muscular activity using the donation arm should be avoided for a short period to prevent the hemostatic seal from breaking loose resulting in additional bleeding. If the donor arm experiences breakthrough bleeding after leaving the donation site, the donor should hold the venipuncture firmly for a few minutes until the bleeding subsides. Donors should refrain from participating in sporting activities using the donation arm for at least 4 hours after donating.

Donor Canteen

Immediately after their donation, donors should be escorted to a canteen area where non-diet drinks and snacks are offered. The items offered in the canteen area are designed to replenish glucose in the donors' bloodstream that may have become depleted during the donation. Donors without symptoms are free to leave the canteen area after 10 to 15 minutes. A bed area should be provided for donors who feel weak where donors can rest until they feel stronger. Supplies should be kept in a handy location close to the canteen area to rebandage arms that experience breakthrough bleeding. However, for safety reasons, the recovery bed should not be kept directly in the canteen area where food and drink are offered.

BIBLIOGRAPHY

Becton C. Drawing blood donor units. Tifton, GA: Personal Interview. November 21, 1997.

Blood donation facts. Available at http://www.net-smart-inc.com/dbqredcross/BloodDonationFacts.cfm. Accessed September 30, 1997.

Blood donation vital to save lives. Available athttp://www.mcg.edu/News/94features/blood donate.html. Accessed September 30, 1997.

BSD 51.110, blood donor interview, processing, and management. Washington DC: American Red Cross, 1996.

Sympatico: HealthWay:Feature:Blood Donation. Available at http://www.sk.sympatico.ca/Contents/HealthyWay/current_tips5.html. Accessed September 30, 1997.

Canine and Feline Phlebotomy

BASICS FOR ANIMAL PHLEBOTOMY

Before attempting to draw any blood from an animal, it is particularly important to approach the animal with a firm yet gentle demeanor. Having a patient's cooperation is vital for relatively painless and careful phlebotomy to occur. Gaining the cooperation of animals for phlebotomy is even more critical in order to obtain a blood sample of sufficient volume and quality for accurate testing purposes. Approaching an animal in a calm friendly manner reassures the animal and makes the animal more likely to be cooperative for phlebotomy. Upset animals are agitated and restless and are unlikely to be obedient even if their master is present. The resulting agitation causes animal movement during phlebotomy unless the animals are restrained for this procedure. Restraint techniques used if an animal seems unlikely to be cooperative and the phlebotomy sites commonly used for canines or felines are discussed below.

If the animal has long or thick hair, clip the hair covering the phlebotomy area. This allows better visualization of the phlebotomy site and gives greater accuracy to the phlebotomist, which results in less trauma to the animal. Repeated tries at phlebotomy will upset most animals causing phlebotomy (and treatment) to be delayed. Once a phlebotomy site has been chosen and hair has been clipped if necessary, prep the animal's skin using an isopropyl alcohol pad. Animals should be muzzled if they threaten to bite during the phlebotomy. Because most peripheral veins in animals are surface veins, the veins are not well-secured in the tissue and tend to roll on needle insertion. For this reason, it is best to begin by inserting the needle just to the side of the selected vein and advance the needle into the vein from the side once the skin has been penetrated. Frontal direct insertion of the needle into this type of vein is possible when performed by an experienced phlebotomist.

Animal phlebotomy can be performed by using a syringe or blood collection tubes. The use of blood collection tubes (e.g., evacuated tubes) greatly simplifies the phlebotomy procedure from fractious animals by freeing another hand to help steady the animal. Gloves are not recommended unless the animal is infected with a disease that is transmissible to humans. Of course, all collection equipment used should by clean and dry before use and discarded into appropriate waste containers after use.

CANINE PHLEBOTOMY

Venipuncture of dogs is usually performed by using the cephalic, jugular, or femoral veins. Blood is usually drawn from the cephalic vein of large breed dogs. The recurrent tarsal vein can also be used for most dogs of other sizes. Clipping the fur of long-haired dogs helps in the visualization of the vein.

The dog that threatens to bite during this procedure can be muzzled for the handler's safety. Dogs can be safely muzzled by placing a long strip of soft cloth under a dog's chin and overlapping the trailing ends over the dog's nose (Fig. 14.1). The ends are then crossed again under the dog's chin and tied

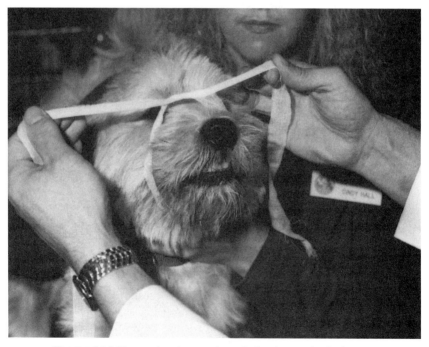

FIGURE 14.1 To muzzle a dog, overlap a cloth strip over the dog's nose.

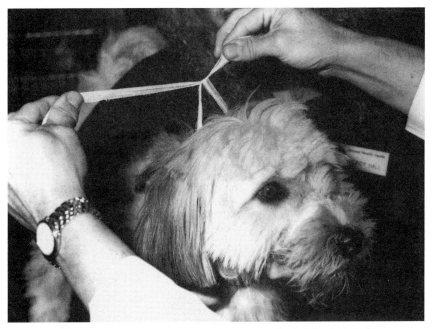

FIGURE 14.2 Tie the trailing cloth strips in a bow behind the dog's head.

behind the animal's head in a bow fashion (Fig. 14.2). Using a bow to secure the ends of the muzzle allows the cloth to secure the animal's closed jaw, yet allows the muzzle to be removed quickly and easily.

Cephalic Vein

To perform phlebotomy from the right cephalic vein, place the dog on its left side on a table. An assistant stands to the left of the dog and restrains the animal by grasping the dog under the chin and around the neck with their right arm and holds the animal close to their body. The assistant's left hand extends the dog's right leg forward for phlebotomy by grasping the right elbow of the dog firmly with their left hand (Fig. 14.3).

The phlebotomist approaches the dog from the right front, grasps the cephalic vein, and rolls it to the side with his/her thumb thus better exposing the cephalic vein. Phlebotomy is performed by inserting the needle between the dog's wrist and elbow (Fig. 14.4). If the animal begins to struggle, the assistant and the phlebotomist maintain control of the animal by pressing it firmly to the table (Fig 14.5).

To perform phlebotomy from the left foreleg, simply reverse the placement instructions given above.

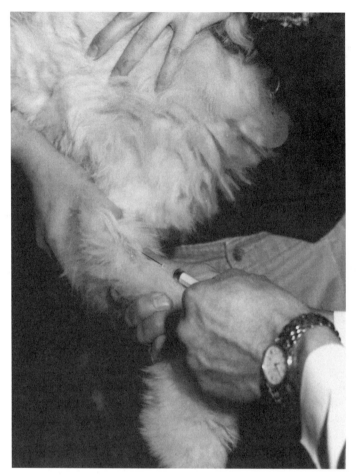

FIGURE 14.3 Phlebotomist extending foreleg in preparation for blood draw.

Jugular Vein

The jugular vein in dogs is easily seen once the dog's head and neck are positioned correctly. The visualization of this large vein can be increased by clipping the hair from this site. This is the most common site for the phlebotomy for small breed dogs. The assistant immobilizes the animal by grasping the dog's forelegs above the elbows with his/her right hand. The left hand of the assistant extends the dog's chin up and back exposing the dog's neck. Often, the position of the dog's head can be slightly turned to bring the jugular vein into better view. Phlebotomists can bring this vein into greater prominence by inserting their thumb into the jugular furrow at the thoracic inlet just prior to phlebotomy.

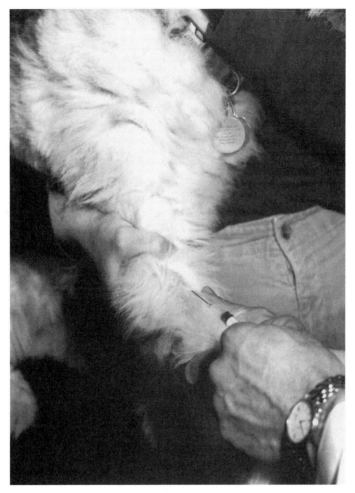

FIGURE 14.4 Insertion of the needle between the dog's wrist and elbow.

Femoral Vein

Drawing blood from the femoral vessel is used more often for obtaining blood from small breed dogs or when larger amounts of blood are needed. This vein is found by placing the dog in a recumbent position and extending a back leg. Using one hand, feel for a pulse in the femoral region of the hip joint. While an assistant controls the dog's movements, carefully puncture the femoral vessel to obtain blood. Since the flow from this vessel is strong, blood is quickly obtained. After phlebotomy has been completed, hold pressure on this site to prevent further bleeding.

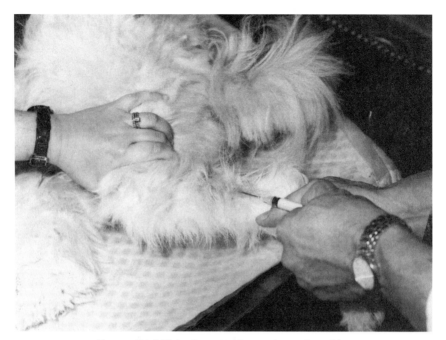

FIGURE **14.5** Maintain control by pressing against table.

Recurrent Tarsal Vein

The recurrent tarsal vein is located on the back legs of animals. This vein is used most often when an animal is unsettled or is upset by being approached from the front. This condition is referred to as being "head-shy" because animals are calmed by being approached from the rear. Because the recurrent tarsal vein is not easily viewed, often the hair covering this site needs to be clipped. To perform phlebotomy using the hindleg of a dog, place the dog on its side opposite of the leg used for phlebotomy. The assistant provides control by pressing on the dog's neck with his/her forearm while grasping the lower rear leg. Another assistant firmly holds the upper rear foreleg above the knee. The upper foreleg is pulled to extension by the phlebotomist. If needed, a tourniquet can be applied to further identify this vein. This site is challenging for inexperienced phlebotomist because this vein is not anchored by tissue and moves easily.

FELINE PHLEBOTOMY

Cats especially need a calm quiet environment with gentle handling in an unhurried manner for successful phlebotomy. Restraint should be gentle yet

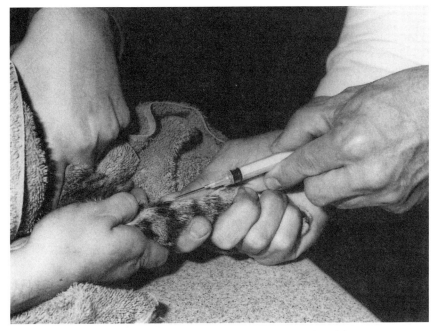

FIGURE 14.6 Cat restrained in towel with limb exposed for phlebotomy.

firm. Often cats can be restrained by being rolled in a towel with the limb for intended phlebotomy exposed (Fig. 14.6). The remaining hindlegs or forelegs should be taped together low enough to cover the claws. Alternately, the cat can be carried under the arm of an assistant whose fingers separate and control the forelegs of the cat. The cat is held snugly against the assistant's body by their elbow pressing the cat against his/her waist and hips. This makes the cat more easily controllable and safer to handle. Common sites for feline phlebotomy are the jugular, cephalic, and femoral veins.

Jugular Vein

The technique for the jugular phlebotomy of cats is very similar to the technique for dogs. The cat is rolled in a towel or placed in a cat bag with the head and neck exposed. A soft cloth muzzle can also be used if necessary. The assistant cradles the cat with one arm holding it next to his/her body. The other hand extends the cats chin up and back exposing the cat's neck. The phlebotomist then locates the jugular vein and proceeds with the venipuncture.

Cephalic Vein

The cephalic vein is exposed by wrapping the cat in a towel with the chosen foreleg exposed. The assistant holds the covered cat closely to his/her body while extending out the foreleg. The worried cat can be calmed by covering its eyes from viewing the phlebotomy procedure with a towel.

Femoral Vein

The femoral vein can be used effectively to obtain blood from a cat, although it is not supported well by subcutaneous tissue, which leads to the frequent formation of hematomas. After clipping the hair from the median side of the leg, the venipuncture site is swabbed with isopropyl alcohol, and the phlebotomy performed. This site is often favored for cat phlebotomy because of the relative ease of locating this prominent vein in cats.

BIBLIOGRAPHY

Benjamin MM. Outline of veterinary clinical pathology. 3rd ed. Ames, IA: Iowa State University Press, 1978.

Dog Owners Guide, Veterinary Technicians. Available at http://www.canismajor. com/dog/vettech.html. Accessed August 13, 1997.

Kirk RW. Handbook of veterinary procedures and emergency treatment. Philadelphia: WB Saunders Co., 1985.

Pratt PW. Medical nursing for animal health technicians. 1st ed. Santa Barbara, CA: American Veterinary Productions, 1985

Veterinary Technicians. Available at http://www. globalx.net/ocd/directions/3213. html. Accessed September 25, 1997.

C H A P T E R **15**

Specimen Collection Other Than Blood

The computer industry coined the phrase: "Garbage in, garbage out". While this is applicable to all types of specimens, it is particularly applicable to specimens other than blood because of the many collection variables that may be introduced. Like blood, other specimens must be collected in appropriate receptacles, properly labeled, and suitably stored if not tested within a short time after collection. In addition, each specimen to be discussed has its own unique collection requirement of which the collector must be aware of and carefully perform. Improperly collected specimens can give erroneous results, which can cause improper patient treatment. Outlined below are procedures for the collection of specimens other than blood that are frequently required for diagnostic or evaluation purposes.

CLEAN-CATCH URINE FOR MICROBIOLOGICAL STUDIES

While the technique of collecting a clean-catch urine specimen is not complex, the possibility of contamination makes it imperative that instructions to the patient be complete and understandable. This will gain the patient's cooperation and thus insure the collection of an acceptable specimen.

Supplies Needed for Each Patient

1. A sterile covered container with an opening large enough for easy collection.
2. Two commercial towelettes containing benzalkonium chloride.

Collection Instructions

FEMALES

1. Supplies should be removed from their packages.
2. The patient should remove undergarments.
3. Next the patient should wash hands with soap and water, rinse, and thoroughly dry the hands with disposable paper towels.
4. The patient should spread the vaginal lips apart. Then using one of the commercial towelettes, cleanse with one wipe in a front to back motion.
5. Properly discard this towelette.
6. Repeat the procedure with the second antiseptic towelette, properly discarding the towelette after use. Instead of antiseptic towelettes, the patient may use gauze pads with soap and water to clean the urethral area. Wet additional gauze pads with water to rinse soap from the area before beginning collection.
7. Continuing to hold the vaginal lips apart, the patient should begin voiding into the commode. Without stopping the urination, the patient should collect a specimen in the sterile container provided. The container should be held with fingers away from its rim and inner surfaces.
8. Avoiding any contact with its inner surfaces, the lid should be securely tightened to prevent leakage.

MALES

1. Supplies should be removed from their packages.
2. The hands should be washed as described in procedure #3 above.
3. The head of the penis (*glans penis*) should be cleansed with a towelette using a front to back motion. Both antiseptic towelettes should be used. If uncircumcised, the patient should completely retract the foreskin. It should be kept retracted throughout the collection procedure. Alternately, soap and water may be used to clean the head of the penis. Rinse soap from the area using clean gauze pads and water.
4. Properly discard the towelettes or gauze pads.
5. The patient should begin voiding into the commode, and then without stopping, collect a remaining portion of the urine into the sterile container provided.
6. During the collection, the sterile container should be held as described in procedure #7 above. The lid should be securely replaced after the sample has been collected without touching the inside.

INFANTS

1. Gently clean the external genitalia.
2. Apply a sterile U-bag over the genitalia, and pull the end of the bag

through a small hole, which has been cut in the crotch of the infant's diaper.

3. After the infant urinates, the bag can be removed and the specimen transferred into a sterile container.

Unless the clean-catch specimen is going to be transported immediately to the laboratory, the specimen should be refrigerated at 4 to 6°C. Alternatively, it may be transferred into a container with boric acid. If this is done, refrigeration is not required. Specimens placed in containers with boric acid cannot be used for a complete urinalysis.

OTHER MICROBIOLOGICAL SPECIMENS

Sputum

Contamination of sputum by upper respiratory tract secretions prevents the acquisition of a clinically relevant specimen. Consequently, the collection of an acceptable sputum sample requires patience and good instruction. It is important that the health care worker assisting in the collection remain with the patient during the entire process. Having the patient gargle with water just before trying to obtain a specimen helps reduce contamination. Removal of any dentures may also be practical. Most patients can produce sputum with a deep cough. Ideally, sputum collection should be done by respiratory therapy; particularly on patients with a nonproductive cough or suspected of having an anaerobic infection. The specimen must be collected in a sterile container with a screw cap and properly identified.

Throat and Nasopharynx

THROAT

It is essential for the diagnosis of upper respiratory infections that the throat swab be well-taken. Collection units with swab and transport media should be used.

1. A bright light should be placed over the shoulder of the health care worker taking the culture. It should be focused into the mouth of the patient.
2. Using a tongue blade, gently depress the tongue.
3. Instruct the patient to breath deeply and say: "ah." This slightly lifts the uvula and helps reduce the gag reflex.
4. Vigorously swab the posterior pharynx (Figure 15.1) using a back and forth sweeping action. Avoid contact with the lateral sides of the mouth, the uvula, tongue, and teeth.
5. Immediately after collecting the specimen, place in the transport medium. Label properly.

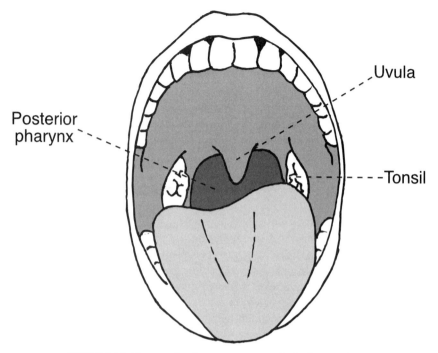

FIGURE 15.1 Diagram showing proper area to obtain throat culture.

NASOPHARYNX

1. Using a calcium alginate swab attached to a flexible wire, gently insert the swab through the nose into the nasopharynx (Figure 15.2).
2. Rotate the swab, then stop, and hold in a still position for 5 to 10 seconds. This allows for additional soaking of secretions onto the swab.
3. Gently remove the swab, and place in a transport medium. Label properly.

Stool

Stools for microbiologic or parasitologic studies should be collected in clean solid containers with leak-proof tops. Avoid Styrofoam and other open containers covered only with aluminum foil. It is recommended that diapers not be submitted. Rather, the specimen should be scraped off the diaper into an acceptable container. Specimens for the identification of parasites should, if possible, be sent as both a fresh specimen and in a fixative solution.

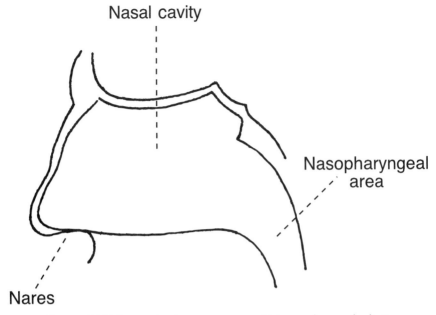

FIGURE 15.2 Diagram showing proper area to obtain nasopharyngeal culture.

Cutaneous Specimens for Fungal Examination

SKIN

1. Cleanse area with 70% alcohol, and let dry.
2. With a scalpel, carefully scrape the peripheral edge of the lesion. This is where the fungus is actively growing.
3. Place scrapings on strong black paper. Fold tightly, and tape at the ends. Place in an envelope for transportation. Label properly.

NAILS

1. Cleanse infected nail(s) with 70% alcohol, and let dry.
2. Scrape nail(s) deeply enough in order to reach recently invaded nail tissue.
3. Discard these initial scrapings.
4. Scrape this underlying nail tissue.
5. Place these scrapings on strong black paper. Fold tightly, and tape the ends. Place in an envelope for transportation. Label properly.

HAIR

Carefully remove infected hair so that the basal portion is attached. Place on strong black paper as previously described. In some cases a Woods lamp (UV light) may be used to select infected hairs. Some dermatophytes cause the infected hairs to fluoresce.

24-HOUR URINE SPECIMEN

An important factor in the collection of a 24-hour urine specimen is to make sure the patient fully understands the process, thus better ensuring cooperation. An incorrect, inadequate, or over-collected specimen will guarantee erroneous results. It is important to go over the collection procedure verbally and also give the patient written instructions.

1. Provide a wide-mouth, plastic container that has a screw lid and is large enough to hold approximately 3 liters.
2. Label the container. If a preservative is required and is added before the collection, warn the patient both verbally and with a label on the container that contact with the preservative could be harmful.
3. Have the patient begin the collection by emptying the bladder at a specified time and discarding this specimen. Instruct the patient to write the date and time the collection was started.
4. Inform the patient to collect *all* voided urine over the next 24-hour period.
5. The patient should conclude the collection exactly 24 hours after it was started by emptying the bladder and adding this to the collection bottle.
6. The urine should stored at 4 to 6°C during the collection period.

SEMEN

1. If the patient is being evaluated for infertility, sexual abstinence should be observed for 3 days before collection.
2. Because of the sensitivity of some of the tests that may be performed on the semen sample, it is best to obtain the specimen at the testing location. The specimen should be collected by masturbation into a pre-warmed (21°C) wide-mouth, sterile, glass or plastic container.
3. Because of personal or religious reasons, collection by masturbation may not be acceptable. In such cases, collection may be by coitus interruptus or using special condoms manufactured specifically for this purpose. *No other type of condom can be used.*
4. If the specimen is collected outside the testing location, the patient should be instructed to note the time the specimen was collected and to get the specimen to the testing location within 1 to 3 hours following collection. During transportation, the specimen should be maintained at body temperature, avoiding exposure to heat and cold.

URINE FOR DRUG SCREEN

Taking illegal drugs causes untold expense in the workplace. Employees under the influence of drugs may miss potentially productive days at work and cause accident rates in the workplace to rise. President Reagan signed Executive Order 12564 establishing the Drug Free Federal Workplace in 1986 to help combat the negative influence of drugs. The order required the Secretary of Health and Human Services to promote technical guidelines for drug testing in the workplace. Most companies now require pre-employment drug testing and random drug testing for established employees to maintain compliance with this Executive Order. Although minor differences in collection requirements exist between certified laboratories and state and federal agencies, the basic principles for the proper collection of urine for drug testing are relatively standard. The following steps generally describe a urine collection procedure.

1. Prior to meeting the donor, check to make sure that all supplies and forms needed for the collection are available. Make sure that a suitable coloring agent such as bluing is visible in the commode in the collection stall.
2. *Supervise the collection of urine from only one donor at a time.*
3. Properly verify the identity of the donor. This can be an official photo ID, identification by a designated representative of the donor's employer, or any identification allowed under a regulatory agency's workplace drug testing program.
4. Ensure that all the information on the control form is correct and complete (i.e., the agency's [employer's] name and address; the medical review officer's [MRO] name and address; the donor's ID number; reason for testing; tests to be performed; and the complete name, address, and telephone number of the collection site).
5. Make a full and careful explanation to the donor about the collection procedure. This includes what personal items can and cannot be taken into the collection stall. Donors must remove outer clothing such as hats, coats, and jackets and leave purses, briefcases, or anything else they are carrying with these garments. Donors may only take their wallets into the collection stall. Donors must not be requested to remove any other articles of clothing or to empty their pockets. *If, however, the collector notices bulging or overstuffed pockets, the collector may request the donor to empty the pockets, display the items, and give an explanation why such items are needed during the collection.* If the donor demands a receipt for any items left outside the stall, the collector must oblige. Lock boxes may be used in which a donor can place personal items such as a wallet or purse. The donor locks the box and takes the key into the collection stall.

6. The collector has the donor wash and dry hands. The donor should not have further access to water.
7. The donor or collector selects a urine collection kit.
8. The donor or collector opens the kit and removes the collection container. The collector retains all items not used directly in the collection.
9. Have the donor go into the stall for the collection. Instruct the donor not to flush the commode or to use any other source of water until the donor has handed the specimen to the collector.
10. After the donor has collected the specimen, it is handed immediately to the collector. *From this point forward, neither the collector, nor the specimen is out of sight of the donor.*
11. The donor is allowed to wash hands.
12. The collector performs the following checks:
    a. The collector observes the specimen for sufficient volume. If the volume is not sufficient, the donor is requested to remain at the collection site, and the donor is given fluids. An attempt is made to collect a new specimen following steps 7 through 11. The insufficient specimen is discarded in a proper manner.
    b. The collector checks the temperature of the specimen using the temperature strip attached to the specimen container (Figure 15.3). The temperature check must be performed within 4 minutes of receiving

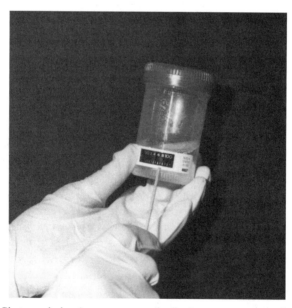

FIGURE 15.3 Photograph showing temperature check using a temperature strip. Note the faint line above pointer is at 97°F, showing that the specimen is within the acceptable range of 90 to 100°F.

the specimen. The acceptable range is 90 to 100°F ± 1.8° of the body temperature. If the temperature is within the 90-to-100°F range, the collector checks the appropriate box on the control form but does not have to record the actual temperature. If the temperature is outside the 90-to-100°F range, the collector records the urine temperature on the control form. The collector then asks the donor if they would like to have a body temperature taken. If the donor agrees and the body temperature is ± 1.8 degrees of the specimen temperature, the specimen is acceptable. The collector notes that the body temperature was taken and records the temperature in the "remarks" section of the control form.

   c. The collector observes the specimen for adulteration such as any unusual color or odor. *If for any reason the collector is sufficiently convinced that the specimen has been adulterated, the collector should notify the donor's agency to see if they wish a specimen collected under direct observation. Do not perform a collection under direct observation without permission from the donor's agency.*

13. If a collection container is used and it is a single specimen collection, the collector pours the minimum required amount into the specimen container. If it is a split-specimen collection, the collector pours at least 30 ml into one specimen container and 15 ml into a second specimen container.

14. The collector now securely places the lid(s) on the specimen container(s). If it is a single specimen collection, the collector now affixes the security seal "A" across the top of the specimen container lid and down the sides of the specimen container (Figure 15.4). If it is a split sample, security seal "A" is affixed to the bottle containing 30 ml and security seal "B" is affixed to the bottle with 15 ml.

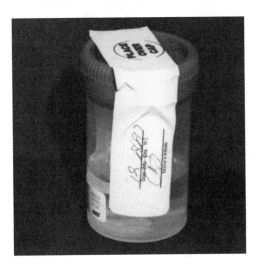

FIGURE 15.4 Photograph showing correct affixation of security seal. Note that the donor has dated and initialed the seal.

15. The donor now initials and dates the seal(s).
16. The donor reads the certification statement in the control form, signs the statement, and completes the information requested.
17. Be sure that the chain of custody section is carefully completed if it is included in the control form. The "Specimen received by" column should have the collector's name and signature. The collector's name and signature should also be in the "Specimen released by" column. Don't forget to date both columns. The collector should print the name of the carrier or shipment provider in the second "Specimen received by" column. Explain the transfer of the specimen from the collection site to the courier or shipment provider by noting: "Specimen to lab" in the second "Purpose of change" column.
18. The collector now fully completes all "Collector" information on the control form.
19. If the control form has a "donor" copy, this is given to the donor. The copies designated for the laboratory are place in the pouch on the tamperproof bag.
20. The specimen (two specimen containers if it is a split sample) is placed in a tamperproof bag, and the bag is sealed (Figure 15.5).
21. The donor is now allowed to leave the collection site.

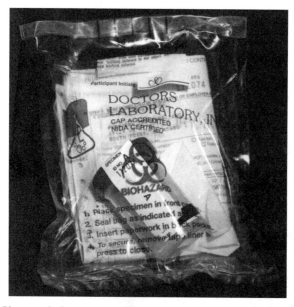

FIGURE 15.5 Photograph showing urine drug screen sample in a sealed tamper-proof bag. Note the donor's initials.

22. The indicated copy of the control form is sent to the MRO if a MRO is designated. If applicable, a copy is sent to the donor's agency, and another copy is retained at the collection site.

In summary, it is the responsibility of the collector to 1) verify the identity of the donor, 2) be responsible for the security of the collection site, 3) ensure the security and integrity of specimens collected, and 4) accurately complete all required documents. In addition, the collector should assure the modesty and privacy of the donor, avoid any remarks of an accusatorial or offensive nature, and supervise the collection of only one donor at a time.

BIBLIOGRAPHY

Bannatyne RM, Clausen C, McCarthy IB. Laboratory diagnosis of upper respiratory infections, Cumitech 10. Washington, DC: ASM Press, 1979.

Baron EJ, Peterson LR, Finegold SM. Diagnostic microbiology. 9th ed. St. Louis, MO: CV Mosby, 1994.

Barry AL, Smith PB, Turch M. Laboratory diagnosis of urinary tract infections, Cumitech 2. Washington, DC: ASM Press, 1975.

Bartlett JG, Brewer NS, Ryan KJ. Laboratory diagnosis of lower respiratory infections, Cumitech 7. Washington, DC: ASM Press, 1978.

Drew DC. Collection steps. The drug free workplace. Available at: http://www.drugfreeworkplace.com. Accessed December 3, 1997.

Koneman FW, Allen SD, Dowell VR Jr, et al. Color atlas and textbook of diagnostic microbiology. 2nd ed. Philadelphia, PA: JB Lippincott Co., 1983.

Laarone DH. Medically important fungi. 3rd ed. Washington, DC: ASM Press, 1995.

Murray PR. ASM pocket guide to clinical microbiology. Washington, DC: ASM Press, 1996.

National Association of Collection Sites. Urine specimen collector's handbook. Alexandria, VA: National Association of Colleciton Sites, 1997.

Weitzman I. ASCP Fall Teleconference Series #8014: the dermatophytes. Chicago, IL: American Society of Clinical Pathologists, November 26, 1996.

Wenk RE. Collection and preservation of timed urine specimens: proposed guideline. Wayne, PA: National Committee for Clinical Laboratory Standards, 1987.

The Electrocardiogram

The electrocardiogram (ECG or EKG) is a graphic record or tracing showing the electric current generated by the various cycles of the heartbeat. This discussion on the ECG will be limited to three areas: the first will give an overview of electrophysiology, the second will give a synopsis of electrocardiography, and the third will cover several prudent practices that should be observed when taking an ECG.

Broadly put, an ECG is a "picture" of the electrical activity of the heart. The body is a good conductor of electricity because fluids in the tissues have a high concentration of ions. Thus, the electric activity generated by the heart is conducted to the body surface and can be recorded as an ECG using an instrument called an electrocardiograph. The honor of being called "The Father of Electrocardiography" is given to Willem Einthoven, a Dutch physiologist. In 1902 he was the first person to record the heart's electric activity in an accurate and reproducible manner. However, the thought that electricity could originate from a biologic source was suggested by the Italian anatomist Luigi Galvani as early as the late 1700s.

OVERVIEW OF ELECTROPHYSIOLOGY

At this point it might be a good idea to re-read the section on the Heart in Chapter 7. There are several important concepts to remember. First, while all the cells in the heart are acting as a single cell or system, they are also acting as two different units—the atria as one unit and the ventricles as another. Second, the heart is innervated by the autonomic nervous system, but it does not initiate contraction. What we think of as the action of the heartbeat is possible because the heart has specialized muscle tissue that generates and distributes the electric impulses that cause the heart to contract. These specialized tissues are the sinoatrial (SA) node, the atrioventricular (AV) node, the AV bundle or bundle of His, and the Purkinje fibers. Third, two types of electrical processes occur during the heartbeat. These are designated as **depolarization** and **repolarization.**

Closely associated with these two types of electrical processes are the chemical elements sodium and potassium (others are involved such as chloride and calcium, but our discussion will be limited to these two.) Both are positively-charged ions and are also known as electrolytes (Fig. 16.1).

- Stimuli originating from the SA node causes the cardiac cells to become permeable to the flow of ions. It is like little pumps in the membranes begin pumping ions either out of or into the cells.
- As more sodium ions are pumped into a cardiac muscle cell, these positive sodium ions, and the positive potassium ions already inside the cell, cause the inside of the cell to become more positive than the outside. This means that the membrane potential has moved toward a more positive value (Fig. 16.2). Thus the cell is **depolarized** or in an *apolarized state.* This action in the flow of sodium ions and the resulting change in membrane potential is called **depolarization.**
- At this time, the cardiac muscle cells become shorter and contract. Depolarization is not, however, the same thing as contraction. Depolarization is an electrical event in which contraction is the expected result.
- After the cell membrane reaches its threshold level, the **cell membrane sodium pumps** slow down and the **cell membrane potassium pumps** begin to rapidly move potassium out of the cell.
- Consequently, there are now fewer positive ions inside the cell; so the membrane potential becomes reversed—moving toward a more negative value. This electrical process is called **repolarization.** The cell is now **polarized** or in a **resting state.**
- Immediately there is a influx of sodium ions back into the cell, and the cycle repeats itself again and again.

SYNOPSIS OF ELECTROCARDIOGRAPHY

When interpreting an ECG, the cardiologist considers several areas, including the heart's rate, rhythm, and axis, and evidence of hypertrophy. The cardiologist does this using different lead positions. To illustrate, if you saw a picture of a house from just one view, let's say the front, your perspective of the house would be very limited. However, if you were able to see several pictures of the house from different angles, you would get a much better idea about its size, configuration, and condition. Similarly, the ECG, using different lead positions, is giving a variety of views of the heart. This information will assist the cardiologist in making an interpretation and diagnosis.

Atoms are electrically neutral because they have the same number of positively-charged protons contained in the nucleus as they do negatively-charged electrons moving around the nucleus. If the atom gains or loses an electron, its overall charge changes and it is called an ion. In the examples below, the sodium has 11 protons. It has given up one electron so that it has only 10 electrons. Because it has one more proton than electrons, it has a positive charge of one or +1. This positively-charged sodium atom is now called a sodium ion, which is noted as Na^+. Likewise, the potassium atom has given up one of its 19 electrons so that now it has only 18. The potassium nucleus contains 19 protons so now its ion also has a positive charge of one (K^+).

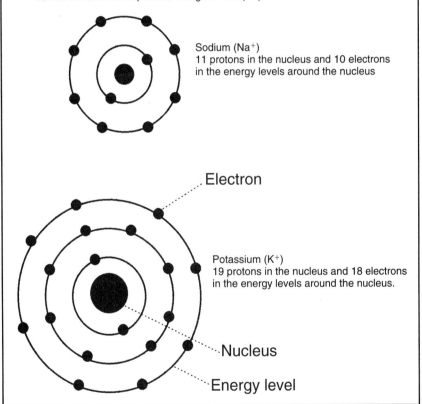

Sodium (Na^+)
11 protons in the nucleus and 10 electrons in the energy levels around the nucleus

Electron

Potassium (K^+)
19 protons in the nucleus and 18 electrons in the energy levels around the nucleus.

Nucleus

Energy level

FIGURE 16.1 Atomic structure of sodium and potassium ions.

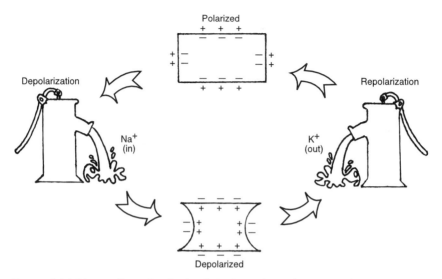

FIGURE 16.2 Diagram illustrating the depolarization and "repolarization" of cardiac muscle brought about by the shifting of ions through the cell walls.

Location and Names of the Monitoring Leads

The 12-lead electrocardiograph is routinely used for diagnostic purposes. The 12 leads are:

Leads I, II, and III

Leads AVR, AVL, and AVF

Leads V_1, V_2, V_3, V_4, V_5, and V_6

The 12 leads look at the heart electrically from different planes in 12 different positions to provide as accurate view of the heart as possible.

Leads I, II, and III are called **bipolar** or **limb** leads. The electrodes are attached to the patient's arms and legs. Each lead records the activity between two different electrodes; one of which serves as the positive, the other as the negative. A third electrode is used as a ground (Table 16.1). The positive is the recording electrode.

The AVR, AVL, and AVF leads (The "A" stands for augmented) are unipolar leads. That is, they use the limbs as the positive or recording electrodes, but use the center of the heart (AV node) as the negative electrode. The last six leads are the **chest,** "**V,**" or **precordial** leads. They are placed on the patient's chest in a semicircle around the heart. As with the augmented leads, the center of the heart (AV node) serves as the negative electrode while each one of the "V" positions is a positive electrode.

Table 16.1. Appendages That Serve as Positive and Negative Poles or Ground for ECG Leads I, II, and III.

Lead	Positive pole	Negative pole	Ground
I	Left arm	Right arm	Right leg
II	Left leg	Right arm	Right leg
III	Left leg	Left arm	Right leg

ECG = electrocardiogram.

Viewing the Heart's Electrical Activity

As stated previously, the ECG looks at the heart electrically from different planes and positions. The electrical relationship of the limb and augmented leads is derived and explained using the Einthoven's triangle (Fig. 16.3). However, in this discussion on the electrical relationships and the areas of the heart that each lead examines, let us pretend that the heart lies within a 360° compass (Fig. 16.4). Lead I is a leftward lead. That is, it records the difference in the electric potential between the negative electrode on the right arm and the positive electrode on the left arm. Thus, it views the heart's electric activity from a vantage point defined as zero degrees (0°). Lead II records the difference in the electric potential between the negative electrode on the right arm and the positive electrode on the left leg. Lead III records the difference

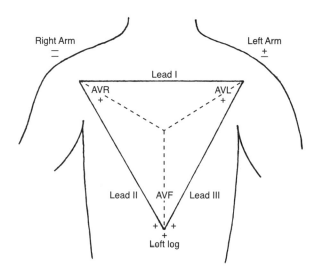

FIGURE 16.3 The Einthoven's triangle.

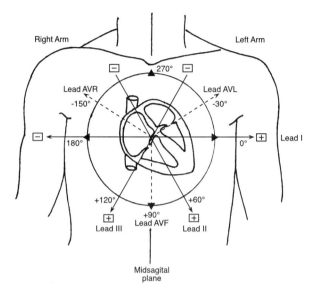

FIGURE 16.4 The electrical relationships and areas of the heart that each lead examines.

between the positive pole on the left leg and the negative pole on the left arm. Leads II and III view the heart's electric activity from a vantage point of +60° and +120°, respectively. The plus sign indicates that the QRS complex (which will be discussed later) is normally in the positive deflection or points upward; a minus sign indicates a downward deflection.

The augmented leads record the difference in the electric potential between the electrodes located on the right arm plus left arm and leg and the center of the heart. These leads view the heart's electrical activity from a vantage point of +90° (AVF), -150° (AVR), and -30° (AVL). These first six leads look at the heart from top to bottom, right and left, and along the frontal plane. Conversely, the chest leads look at the heart from different positions in a horizontal plane or cross section as demonstrated in Figure 16.5.

The Electrocardiogram Wave

The purpose of the ECG is to give a means whereby a clinician may visually assess the pattern of the electric wave as it progresses through the heart. Abnormalities such as irregular rhythms, enlargement of the heart, electrolyte imbalance, and coronary heart disease may be determined by evaluating the tracings or patterns made of the heart's electrical activity. In addition, the ECG may be used to monitor the side effects of drugs that might affect the heart and to check the function of artificial pacemakers. Although the ECG is a valuable diagnostic tool, it must be understood that it cannot serve

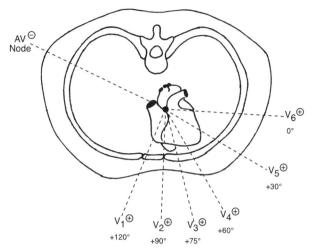

FIGURE 16.5 Cross section of how the chest leads look at the heart.

as a crystal ball. The ECG can show the condition of the heart at the time the ECG is taken, but it cannot predict the future.

The ECG Graph Paper

Continuous ECG signals may be followed on an oscilloscope (a monitor that looks like a television screen), but more familiar is the ECG done using a 12-lead machine that must be removed from the patient after the tracings are made. Familiar too are the hard copies of the tracings using a standardized graph paper, which is illustrated in Figure 16.6.

Note that the graph paper is composed of two size squares. The small squares measure 1 mm by 1 mm, and the larger squares measure 5 mm by 5 mm. The horizontal plane of the ECG measures time, and the vertical plane measures voltage. Each small square horizontally represents 0.04 second of time, and each large square represents 0.2 second of time. Vertically each small square represents 0.1 mV and each large square 0.5 mV. Because the graph paper moves at a standardized speed in the electrocardiograph, the clinician is able to utilize the information given above to determine, for example, cardiac conductivity and heart rate.

The P-Q-R-S-T-U Cycle

The ECG waves have been labeled P, Q, R, S, and T (throughout the discussion in this section please refer to Figure 16.6). These waves represent the depolarization and repolarization of different areas of the heart. Their deflec-

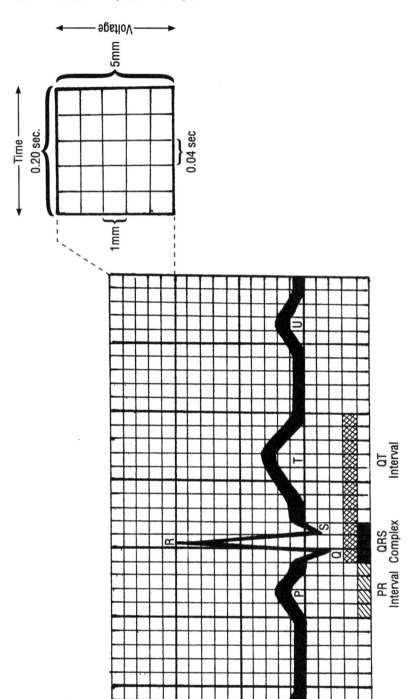

FIGURE 16.6 ECG tracing on standardized graph showing major waveforms. Note that the time in seconds is measured on the horizontal axis while voltage in millimeters is measured on the vertical axis.

tion depends on the lead (i.e., I, II, III, AVF, AVL, AVR, etc.) and the area of the heart the lead is focusing on.

The first wave in the cycle is the P wave. It represents the depolarization of the atria. Actually, excitation starts at some point before the P wave (as represented by the flat isoelectric line), but the electric activity is too small to measure. The area between the P wave and the R wave is called the P-R segment and is the period of atrial repolarization. The Q, R, and S waves are called the QRS interval and represent ventricular depolarization. From the S wave to the end of the T wave represents repolarization of the ventricular musculature.

RECOMMENDED ELECTROCARDIOGRAM TECHNIQUES

A variety of manufacturers and models of electrocardiographs makes it impractical to outline in detail the procedure for performing an ECG. All ECGs have similar basic components: 1) electrodes or sensors, 2) lead wires, 3) an amplifier, and 4) chart recorder. Additional components are required for those ECG machines that are used for continuous monitoring. The following are some prudent practices that should be observed regarding ECG procedures:

- The lead wires should periodically be disinfected by rubbing the wires with a cloth moistened with formaldehyde or an approved disinfectant.
- On models that have nondisposable electrodes, the electrodes should be polished on a regular basis to ensure good conductivity. These electrodes should also be disinfected.
- The skin should be well cleansed for electrodes to have good contact. Oils, dirt, or perspiration will prevent the electrodes from making good contact with the skin resulting in poor conductivity.
- Place the electrodes as much as possible in hairless areas. Remove extra hair if necessary.
- When applying disposable electrodes, avoid touching the sticky side. After application, smooth the electrode on the skin to make sure there is good contact.
- If the disposable electrodes have tabs, make sure that the tabs point toward the heart. That is, the tabs should point downward on the arms and chest and upward on the legs.
- Make sure that electrodes used on the arms and legs are not positioned over a bony area. Place them on a fleshy part of the limb.
- Be certain that the correct lead wire is connected to the proper electrode. Most lead wires are both color-coded and monogrammed. The American Hospital Association color code is as follows:

Monogram	Body Connection	Location	ECG Connection
RL	Green	Right leg	Green
LL	Red	Left leg	Red
RA	White	Right arm	White
LA	Black	Left arm	Black
V_1	Brown	Chest	Red
V_2	Brown	Chest	Yellow
V_3	Brown	Chest	Green
V_4	Brown	Chest	Blue
V_5	Brown	Chest	Orange
V_6	Brown	Chest	Purple

- When connecting the lead wires, avoid large loops. Have the wires lay flat against the patient and follow the contour of the patient's body.
- Be certain of the proper placement of the chest electrodes or sensors (Fig. 16.7). When recording ECGs from pediatric patients, the V_4 electrode is often transposed to the 5th intercostal space on the right side of the sternum.

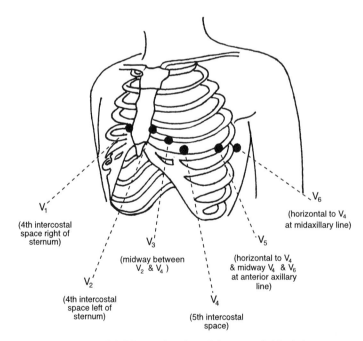

FIGURE 16.7 Proper location of the precordial lead sites.

BIBLIOGRAPHY

Bean DY. Introduction to ECG interpretation. Rockville, MD: Aspen Publishers, Inc., 1987.

Catalano JT. Guide to ECG analysis. Philadelphia, PA: JB Lippincott, 1993.

Davis GP Jr, Parks E. The heart: the living pump. New York: Torstar Books, 1984.

Grauer K. A practical guide to ECG interpretation. St. Louis, MO: Mosby YearBook, Inc., 1992.

Jenkins D. A brief history of electrocardiography, 1997. Available at: http://home-pages.enterprise.net/djenkins/ecghist.html. Accessed August 3, 1997.

Operating instructions: E350i interpretive electrocardiograph. Milton, WI: Burdick, Inc., 1993.

Urosevich RB, McVan B, eds: Reading EKG's correctly. 2nd ed. Springhouse, PA: Springhouse Corp., 1984.

Quality Control for Point-of-Care Testing

DEFINITION OF QUALITY CONTROL

In today's lexicon there are a number of terms that seem to be ubiquitously associated with quality medical care. These terms are: *quality control, quality assurance, continuous quality improvement,* and *quality management.* Definitions of the terms tend to overlap, and attempts to differentiate them result in very tedious explanations. Consequently, the scope of this chapter will be limited to that area that the person doing point-of-care testing is most concerned with—*quality control.*

Quality control (QC) can be defined as a system that is used to maintain a determined level of accuracy and precision as applied to analytical analysis. Its primary purpose is to ensure the reported results of any patient laboratory testing are correct. As noted in previous chapters, QC applies not only to the direct examination of the specimen, but also to how the specimen was attained. To fully apprehend QC, there are two terms that must be understood. These terms are *precision* and *accuracy.*

Let's say that you shoot three arrows at a target, with your objective being to hit the bull's-eye each time. Looking at the first target (Fig. 17.1) you will see that not once did you hit the bull's-eye, nor did you get any of your arrows near each other. In other words, you were neither accurate (you didn't hit the bull's-eye) nor were you precise (the arrows were all over the target). You try again. This time (Fig. 17.2) you got all of your arrows to hit the target in the upper right area. You were very precise. You got your arrows to hit near the same spot every time, but you were not accurate. You still didn't hit the bull's-eye. You try once more. This time you get all of your arrows to hit the bull's-eye. (Fig. 17.3) Not only are you now precise in your shooting, but you are also accurate. Precise means that you are consistent with your results. You are getting similar outcomes time after time. Accuracy means that those outcomes are actual. By applying QC, you monitor test results using a control material

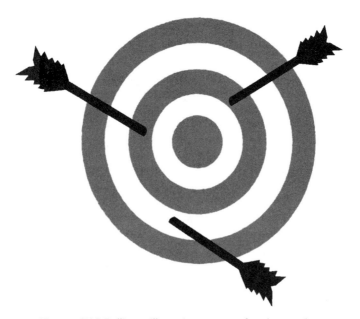

FIGURE 17.1 Bull's-eye illustrating concept of random results.

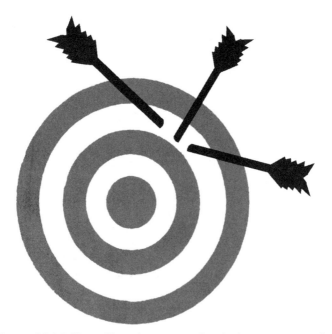

FIGURE 17.2 Bull's-eye illustrating concept of precise but inaccurate results.

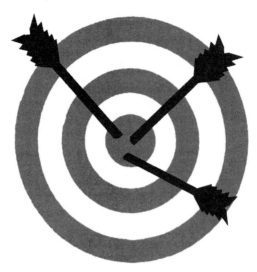

FIGURE 17.3 Bull's-eye illustrating concept of both precise and accurate results.

in order to measure and control the testing system. This is so that you can be confident that outcomes from that testing system are true or accurate.

CONTROL MATERIALS

To achieve the statistical requirements of quality control, QC programs require the same sample to be tested everyday that testing is done. This type of sample is usually purchased and is called a *control*. Most controls use a human base to ensure the analytes being tested parallel human ranges. Many human blood samples are pooled together by manufacturers to help create the large volume needed for a *lot number* of control. To help ensure the safety of those performing patient testing, most manufacturers produce lot numbers of control material that test negative for the human immunodeficiency virus (HIV) and hepatitis B virus (HBV). Manufacturers place the same batch or lot number of control material into small vials. This allows only a small portion of the control to be handled while the remainder is stored until needed. The manufacturer will print on the vial the way the control should be stored. The storage instructions should be followed meticulously to ensure the stability of the control material.

Regardless of the laboratory test, whether it be chemistry or blood banking, controls must share certain similarities to the type of human sample whose accuracy is being monitored by QC. For hematology analyzers, controls need to have the same consistency and color as that found in human blood. Likewise, serum controls need to have similar amounts of chemicals close to those found in human serum. QC of potassium is not accomplished when the potassium in a control far exceeds the level found in humans. If a control contains a range of potassium that mirrors the range of that found in humans, it appropriately "controls" potassium testing.

Before controls can be run, every testing instrument must first be *calibrated* for use. Calibration requires *standards,* or testing solutions with known values. The instrument is calibrated when it accurately measures the amount of analyte in the standard. This allows every unknown patient sample or control to be analyzed from a measured starting point. Standards *should not be run as daily controls* because they do not measure or "control" other variables in the testing process such as operator technique or sample appropriateness.

QUALITY CONTROL FUNDAMENTALS

The basic purpose of QC is to monitor and control analytic error (systematic and/or random) when performing a testing procedure. The bottom line being: is the result of the test procedure good—I *can* accept it with absolute certainty. Or, is the result uncertain—I *can't* accept it with absolute certainty.

There is no one QC format that is appropriate or practical for every testing situation; nor is there one perfect QC system that will detect every error. Many rules and viewpoints regarding QC have either shifted or emerged as technology has changed. The QC schemes discussed in this chapter are simply to illustrate how QC can be applied toward the total quality management of point-of-care testing.

Random and Systematic Errors

What type of problems are monitored by QC? Faulty performances that cause an error in test results fall into two large categories. Sources of incorrect testing data are: *random error* and *systematic error*. Both types of errors must be investigated and resolved for accurate and precise testing. Random error occurs because of extremely small variables in testing that are not easily managed, such as strictly defined sample size or exact pipette delivery. Random error affects the *precision* of a test. Random error also occurs when an inappropriately collected specimen is used for testing.

Systematic error occurs when a process alters the testing process, which causes all results to be biased. Here, the entire process of testing is changed by an event that alters the *accuracy* of the testing process. For example, when improper standards for calibration are used or a dirty lens is present in a measuring device, a systematic error may be expected. In these cases, the instrument is deviating all of its measurements, both patients and controls. The deviation of control values causes the mean value to change, but the deviation of patient values causes inaccurate test results. Consequently, any change in the statistical mean is an indication of a systematic error and must be investigated.

Quality Control Documentation and Interpretation

The documentation of control results and the daily observation and assessment of that documentation is a must for a good QC program. In this section, we will give an overview of some of the ways to document and assess your QC results. Before beginning, however, there are a minimal number of basic terms, or concepts, that *must* be understood. These include *mean, standard deviation (SD), Gaussian curve,* and *Levey-Jennings chart.*

The *mean* is simply an average of all the data points. Let's say that you performed 100 glucose determinations on a known control sample. The addition of the results of all the tests divided by 100, the number of tests done, would give you the mean or average. The mathematical formula for determining the mean is:

$$Mean = \frac{Sum\ of\ the\ results\ of\ all\ the\ tests}{Number\ of\ tests}$$

The mean is used to detect systematic errors.

Now suppose we took the results of the 100 glucose determinations and plotted them on an X–Y-axis with the Y-axis being the number of tests and the X-axis being the glucose results. More than likely a configuration would be produced that looks very similar to the one illustrated in Figure 17.4. This is called a *histogram*. A histogram is a graph or plot that lets you see how many times a certain event occurred. Statisticians use the term *frequency distribution* to describe a histogram. If we then draw a line from the lowest to the highest numbers in our data, the result would be a curve that looks like the outline of a bell. (Fig. 17.5). This is known as the *Gaussian curve* or more popularly as a *bell-shaped curve*. Note in Figure 17.6 that the curve is divided into six equal sections. Each of these sections is a *SD*. In the middle of these six sections is the *mean*. The shape of the Gaussian curve in Figure 17.6 is for

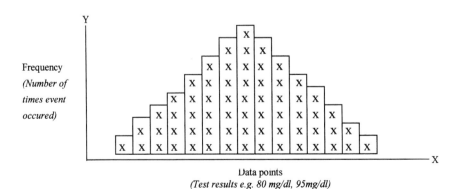

FIGURE 17.4 A histogram is a graph of frequency distribution.

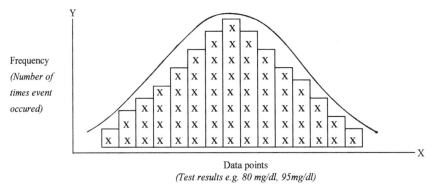

FIGURE 17.5 Development of a Gaussian curve from a histogram.

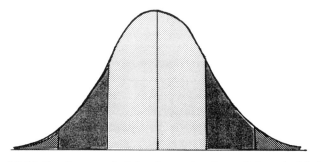

FIGURE 17.6 A Gaussian curve depicting the equal sections called standard deviations.

a normal distribution. Normal distribution denotes that most of the data are close to the average or mean with very few of the data points being at one extreme or the other. If the data points are not close to the mean, the mean the Gaussian curve can acquire other configurations, but that is beyond the scope of this discussion.

The SD is an analytic method used to determine the scatter of results around the mean. Most QC programs are based on the supposition that the majority of test results will fall into a normal Gaussian curve. As you can see in Figure 17.7, approximately 99% of all test results will fall within 3 SD (± 3SD), 95% within 2 SD (± 2SD), and 68% within 1 SD (± 1SD).

To state in very cursory terms, statisticians have determined that values no greater than plus or minus 2 SD represent measurements that are more closely near the true value than those that fall in the area greater than ± 2SD.

As stated previously, documentation and evaluation of QC on a daily basis are vital. One of the most commonly used methods for QC documentation is the *Levey-Jennings Chart*. Its usual configuration is to have the days of the month plotted on the X-axis and the control observations plotted on the Y-

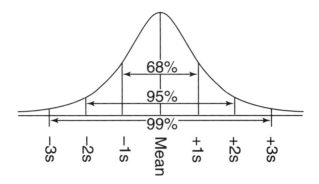

FIGURE 17.7 The Gaussian curve in this figure is one for a normal distribution. Most quality control programs are based on the supposition that values fall into normal distribution and that 95% of all those values will be within $+/-$ 2 standard deviations.

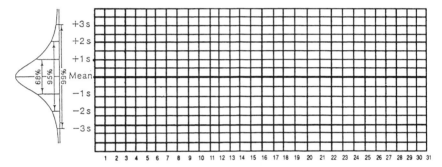

FIGURE 17.8 A typical Levey-Jennings chart used for plotting control data. The days of the month are on the X-axis and the control values on the Y-axis. The Gaussian curve is included to show the correlation of the curve to the chart.

axis. Figure 17.8 shows a typical Levey-Jennings Chart. At its left is the Gaussian curve turned on its side to show the correlation of the curve to the Chart.

By observing the data plotted on the Levey-Jennings chart, we can deduct that the test results are in control and accurate. Or we can deduct that the test results were not in control and consequently unacceptable. However, it is possible to infer that a run is bad when it actually is good and vice versa that a run is good when it is really unacceptable. The important thing is to have an error-detecting scheme that will keep false-accepts and false-rejects low. Use of the Westgard and Cumulative Summation Rules are two QC programs that can help you do this.

WESTGARD RULES

In 1981, James Westgard and his associates developed a multi-rule procedure for interpreting control data. Since then, a number of sophisticated QC schemes or analogues based on this multi-rule logic have evolved. To show how the Westgard Rules may be applied in QC, three of the most common rejection limits are used. Their adaptation to the Levey-Jennings Plot is also illustrated.

1$_{3s}$

This Westgard rule, abbreviated 1$_{3s}$, states that if one of the controls is greater than ± 3 SD, then the patient results would possibly not be true. This is because either a random error or a very large systematic error has occurred. Thus, the run should be rejected. This rule is illustrated in Figure 17.9, which shows two Levy-Jennings plots. The top chart is for the "Normal" control; the bottom chart plots the "Elevated" control. On the 13th day of the month (as noted by the arrow) the elevated control was greater than + 3 SD from the mean. Thus, rule 1$_{3s}$ applies, and the run is rejected. Troubleshooting must be performed before further testing can be performed. This will be discussed under *Systematic Troubleshooting*.

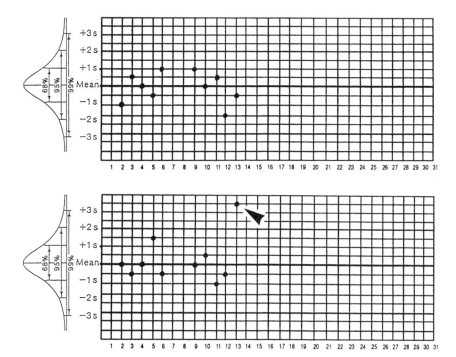

FIGURE 17.9 Levey-Jennings plots illustrating the Westgard Rule 1$_{3s}$. Note that the 13th of the month the elevated control (bottom chart) was greater than +/− 3 standard deviations from the mean.

2_{2s}

Using this rule, if two or more controls are greater than ± 2 SD from the mean on the same day of testing, then the run must be rejected. If this circumstance occurs, it is suggestive of a systematic error. The Levey-Jennings plots on the 13th day for both the normal and elevated controls (Fig. 17.10) show greater than 2SD. Once again, troubleshooting must be performed before further testing can be performed.

4_{1s}

This rule is a bit more complicated and requires more than a glance observation for application. It essentially has two parts. The first part (Fig. 17.11) states that a run is to be rejected if on that day, plus the 3 testing days just prior, the control values were beyond 1 SD. In other words, the control values were beyond 1 SD for 4 consecutive days. The second part of this rule asserts that a run must be rejected if on that day plus the 5 testing days just prior,

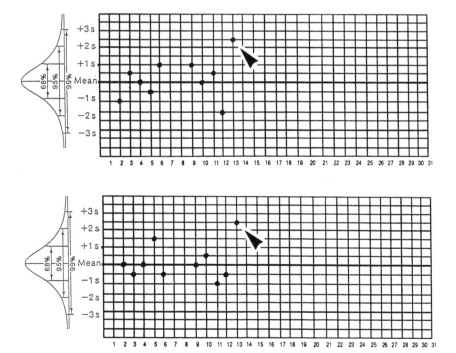

FIGURE 17.10 Levey-Jennings plots illustrating the Westgard Rule 2_{2s}. On the 13th of the month both controls were greater than +2 standard deviations from the mean. Had only one of the controls been greater than +/− 2 standard deviations and not both, the run would have been accepted as in control.

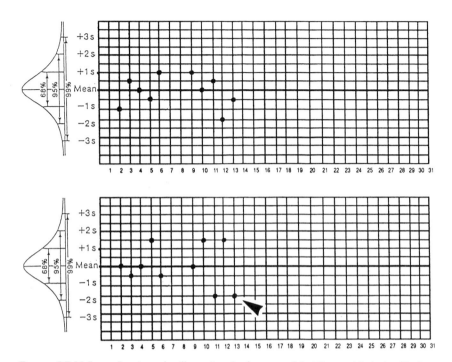

FIGURE 17.11 Levey-Jennings plot illustrating the first part of the Westgard Rule 4_{1S}. Notice that the elevated control on the 10th, 11th, and 12th were greater than $+/-$ 2 standard deviations from the mean. The control was again greater than -2 standard deviation on the 13th, resulting in the testing procedure being of control.

the control values were on the same side of the mean (Fig. 17.12). Continuous plots on one side of the mean is called a *shift*. It could be caused by a number of things including introduction of a new lot number of reagents or control. Regardless, both parts of the rule reflect a systematic error, and troubleshooting must be done before testing can be resumed.

CUMULATIVE SUMMATION RULE

Like the Westgard Rules, the Cumulative Summation Rule (cusum) or Limit has different approaches. The example given is more sensitive to systematic than random error. Nevertheless, it does provide a relatively uncomplicated means to warn of impending problems in the testing process. Figure 17.13 is an illustration of a type of worksheet that can be used to calculate and record the cusum limit (CL). This worksheet will be used in the example, and you will need to refer to Figure 17.14 throughout the discussion. A Levey-Jennings plot has been included so you can correlate it with the cusum values.

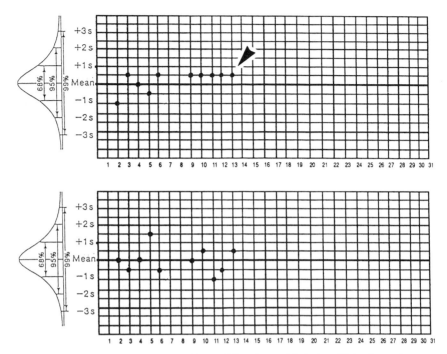

FIGURE 17.12 An illustrates the second part of the Westgard Rule 4_{1S}. All the data points were plotted on the same side of the mean for 6 consecutive days in the normal control.

Note that the right side of the worksheet is used to determine the mean, SD, coefficient of variation (CV), and CL. Using the *sum of results* and the *sum of squared differences* from the mean obtained from control results performed during the month of February, the mean and SD are calculated. The new Normal Glucose Control mean is 95 mg/dl with a ± 1.4 SD. To determine the CL, the SD is multiplied by 2.7. The CL for March is ± 4.0. Some rounding up has been done in all the calculations.

Starting with March 6th, the normal glucose control read 94 mg/dl. Since 94 is less than 95 (the mean), the *difference from the mean* is −1. In the next column the difference is squared. The sign is not significant when squaring a number so the result is $1 \times 1 = 1$. The last column is the *cusum value*. Here the sign is significant. The cusum value was +1 the previous day (March 5th). Today, March 6th, the value was calculated to be −1. Thus −1 from +1 equals 0.

On March 9th, glucose testing was performed and the normal control result was 93. This time the cusum value is −2 since the cusum value for the previous testing period was zero (−2 + 0 = −2). On March 10th the normal control was 94. The cusum value is −1 by reason that 94 is one less than 95. Since the day before, the cusum value was a −2 and they are of a like sign, the two must

Control:_____

Lot #:_____

Test _____

Expiration Date of Control: _____

Dates this Q.C. covers:_____

Daily Results	Difference From Mean	Squared Difference From Mean	Cusum
1. _____	_____	_____	_____
2. _____	_____	_____	_____
3. _____	_____	_____	_____
4. _____	_____	_____	_____
5. _____	_____	_____	_____
6. _____	_____	_____	_____
7. _____	_____	_____	_____
8. _____	_____	_____	_____
9. _____	_____	_____	_____
10. _____	_____	_____	_____
11. _____	_____	_____	_____
12. _____	_____	_____	_____
13. _____	_____	_____	_____
14. _____	_____	_____	_____
15. _____	_____	_____	_____
16. _____	_____	_____	_____
17. _____	_____	_____	_____
18. _____	_____	_____	_____
19. _____	_____	_____	_____
20. _____	_____	_____	_____
21. _____	_____	_____	_____
22. _____	_____	_____	_____
23. _____	_____	_____	_____
24. _____	_____	_____	_____
25. _____	_____	_____	_____
26. _____	_____	_____	_____
27. _____	_____	_____	_____
28. _____	_____	_____	_____
29. _____	_____	_____	_____
30. _____	_____	_____	_____
31. _____	_____	_____	_____

Sum of Results   Sum of Squared Differences From Mean

A. $\text{MEAN} = \dfrac{\text{SUM OF RESULTS}}{\text{N}} = \_\_\_\_$

N = NUMBER OF DAILY RESULTS

B. $\text{SD} = \sqrt{\dfrac{\text{SUM OF SQUARED DIFFERENCES FROM MEAN}}{\text{N} = 1}}$

$\text{SD} = _____$

C. $\text{SD} \times 2 = 2 \text{ STANDARD DEVIATIONS}$

D. $\text{CV (\%)} = \dfrac{\text{SD}}{\text{MEAN}} \times 100$

$\text{CV} = _____$

E. $2.7 \times \text{SD} = \text{CUSUM LIMIT (CL)}$

$\text{CL} = _____$

FIGURE 17.13 Sample worksheet that can be used to calculate the cusum limit.

be added together. Resulting in a cusum value of −3. This value is near the CL of ± 4.0 and should serve as a warning to initiate corrective action. For purpose of example, this warning will be ignored. On the next day, March 11th, the normal control again reads 94 mg/dl with a cusum value of −1. Adding this to the −3 of the previous day, the CL of ± 4.0 has now been reached and the glucose testing procedure is "out of control." Once the calculated CL has been reached the patient test results cannot be accepted as accurate. It is important to daily observe any trends in the cusum values so that corrective action can be taken long before the limit is reached. Looking at the Levey-Jennings chart it will be noticed that the plots correspond with the Westgard Rule 4_{1s}.

SYSTEMATIC TROUBLESHOOTING

Problems are inevitable in QC. Some problems affecting QC can be avoided, such as performing regularly scheduled cleaning and other maintenance of

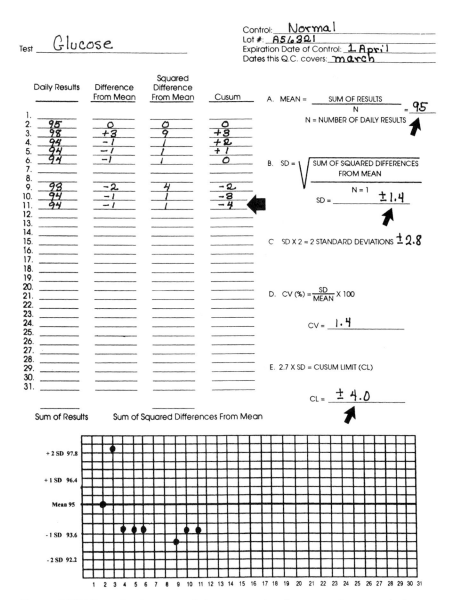

FIGURE 17.14 Example using a normal glucose control to demonstrate how to apply the cusum limit to a quality control program. Refer to text for details.

equipment. Other errors happen suddenly and require immediate action to resolve an analysis that is "out of control."

Accurate and precise measurement can usually be restored by the following steps when QC shows an analysis is "out of control":

1. Rerun the control that is out-of-range. Random errors in sampling may be resolved by simply running the test again using the same control and a fresh testing device. If the result is still unacceptable, the next troubleshooting step should be followed.
2. Make certain all lot numbers and expiration dates of reagents and controls used in the testing process are current. Check the recommended storage conditions.
3. Run the control using a new unopened bottle of control. Improper storage may have accelerated the deterioration of the original control or the testing material may have expired. If these actions do not solve the problem, step #4 should be followed.
4. Review calibration of the test instrument. What was the date of the last calibration? Test instruments need to be calibrated according to the manufacturer's instructions or more frequently if necessary. Federal requirements call for analytic tests to be recalibrated at least every 6 months to verify the accuracy of the testing procedure. If QC results using the old and new controls are not acceptable after recalibration, follow step #5.
5. Call the test manufacturer for advice. Manufacturers have additional information that may help resolve QC problems. Specimens should be stored properly for later testing if the problem cannot be resolved.

BIBLIOGRAPHY

Cembrowski GS, Carey RN. Laboratory quality management QC↔QA. Chicago, IL: ASCP Press, 1989.

Herndon LH. Finding the target: basic quality control for physician office laboratory. Knoxville, TN: American Association of Physician Office Laboratories, RCFA Physician Managers, Inc.

Herring K, McLellan W, Plaut D. QC and new technology: do the old rules still apply. Total quality management, point-of-care testing III. Medical Laboratory Observer 1993;25(95)(Suppl):7.

Moran RF. QC overview. Norwood, MA: Ciba Corning Diagnostics Corp., 1995.

Niles R. Statistics every writer should know: standard deviation. Available at http://www.probe.net/%7Eniles/stdev.html. Accessed on August 9, 1996.

Plaut D, Condiff H. Intra-laboratory quality control. Miami, FL: Baxter Diagnostics, Inc., 1993.

APPENDICES

Appendices

SOURCES FOR EDUCATIONAL MATERIAL

Below is a limited list of resources for educational materials that are suitable for both primary and continuing education. Most distributors of phlebotomy and point-of-care testing supplies and equipment will send printed or video materials regarding their products for distribution or display. In addition, the Internet has an enormous amount of information dealing with subjects related to phlebotomy, infection control, drug screen collection, and quality assurance.

1. *American Society of Clinical Pathologists*
   2100 West Harrison Street
   Chicago, IL 60612-3798
   Telephone (800) 621-4142
   The American Society of Clinical Pathologists (ASCP) has produced a number of excellent videotapes. "Blood Collection: The Pediatric Patient" provides information about performing heelsticks, fingersticks, and venipunctures using a butterfly needle. "Blood Collection: The Routine Venipuncture" demonstrates the routine venipuncture based on National Committee for Clinical Laboratory Standards (NCCLS) and Occupational Safety and Health Administration (OSHA) standards. "Blood Collection: Special Procedures" covers blood cultures, type and crossmatch, special transport, cold agglutinins, the modified Ivy Bleeding time, therapeutic drug monitoring, and glucose tolerance testing. "Blood Collection: The Difficult Draw" discusses the collection of blood from patients in emergency departments, patients receiving treatment, and patients with physical or medical conditions that make blood collection difficult. Details that are discussed for each procedure include site selection and preparation, patient identification, equipment used, and procedure and quality assurance considerations. Videotapes on laboratory safety and infection control and the OSHA recommendations for the prevention of bloodborne pathogens are also available.

2. *Becton Dickinson Media Center*
1 Becton Drive, MC304
Franklin Lakes, NJ 07417-1884
Telephone: (800) 255-6334
   The Becton Dickinson Media Center has a number of videotapes dealing with specimen collection, transportation, and handling plus laboratory safety.

3. *Educational Materials for Health Professionals, Inc.*
607 Wateviliet Avenue
Dayton, OH 45420
Telephone: (937) 254-0990
   Educational Materials for Health Professionals, Inc., has several self-instructional units that are suitable for the patient care technician. At present, all are available in spiral book form, some with 35mm slides. There are self-evaluation questions throughout each unit. Thus, the student can immediately review those sections not understood, rather than wait until the post-test to discover any deficiencies.

4. *Elektro Assemblies, Inc.*
522 N. W. Sixth Avenue
Rochester, MN 55901
Telephone (800) 533-1558
   Elektro Assemblies, Inc., manufactures an inexpensive phlebotomy training device called the *Veni-Dot*. The simulation to an actual arm and veins is excellent. It is portable, easy to assemble, simple to use, and easily stored.

5. *National Committee for Clinical Laboratory Standards*
940 West Valley Road, Suite 1400
Wayne, PA 19087-1898
Telephone: (610) 688-0100
   National Committee for Clinical Laboratory Standards offers several videotapes and publications dealing with specimen collection, handling, processing, evaluation, and laboratory safety.

5. *Southern California Phlebotomy Training*
23010 Lake Forest Drive, Suite 165
Laguna Hills, CA 92653
Telephone: (714) 362-1634
   The Southern California Phlebotomy Training has several training booklets available on subjects relating to phlebotomy procedures and safety.

6. *American Association of Physician Office Laboratories*
P. O. Box 23527
Knoxville, TN 37933-1527
Telephone: (800) 470-9605
   American Association of Physician Office Laboratories offers self-instructional courses on medical terminology, OSHA compliance, quality

control, specimen collection, tuberculosis, and others. Their newsletter is a source of practical information. Training courses offered by other professional organizations may also be listed.

7. *National Association of Collection Sites*
   1600 Duke Street, Suite 220
   Alexandria, VA 22314
   Telephone: (800) 355-1257
   National Association of Collection Sites is strongly committed to the training of individuals associated with drug and alcohol screening collection.

8. *ABP, Inc.*
   51097 Bittersweet Road
   P. O. Box 127
   Granger, IN 46530
   ABP, Inc., publishes a training and review manual on electrocardiography.

PHLEBOTOMY CERTIFYING AGENCIES

1. *American Association of Allied Health Professionals, Inc. (AAAHP)*
   Atrium Executive Center
   80 Orville Drive
   Bohemia, NY 11716
   Telephone: (516)244-1523

   Frequency of examination: Varies with need; the AAAHP has a reclamation program that requires 1 or more years experience as a full-time phlebotomist and a proficiency evaluation administered by the phlebotomist's supervisor.

   Examination format: Multiple choice, true/false, matching, plus proficiency evaluation

   Eligibility routes: Completion of at least 200 hours of an approved training course

   Certification: AAAHP

   Recertification: Recertification yearly by 12 contact hours of continuing education

   The AAAHP also certifies clinical medical assistants and ECG technicians.

2. *American Medical Technologists (AMT)*
   710 Higgins Road
   Park Ridge, IL 60068
   Telephone: (847) 823-5169

   Frequency of examination: Twice per year at designated locations and as needed at ABHES accredited schools

Examination format: Multiple choice
Eligibility Routes: Six months work experience
                    OR
            Graduate of a phlebotomy course given in an accredited school or program
Certification: RPT (AMT)
Recertification: Certification must be renewed yearly. At least 5 contact hours each year of continuing education is encouraged but not required.

3. *American Society of Clinical Pathologists (ASCP)*
Board of Registry
2100 West Harrison Street
Chicago, IL 60612-3798
Telephone: (800) 621-4142

Frequency of examination: Four times per year; given only in designated cities
Examination format: Multiple choice
Eligibility routes: High school diploma or equivalent and completion of a NAACLS approved program within the last 5 years
                    OR
            High school diploma or equivalent and completion of an acceptable structured phlebotomy program
                    OR
            High school diploma or equivalent and 1 year of full-time work experience in phlebotomy within the last 5 years
                    OR
            High school diploma and successful completion of RN, LPN, or other accredited allied health professional/occupational education and phlebotomy training
Certification: PBT (ASCP)
Recertification: Once certified, recertification is not required.

4. *American Society of Phlebotomy Technicians (ASPT)*
P. O. Box 1831
Hickory, NC 28603
Telephone: (704) 322-1334

Frequency of examination: Varies with need; if application approved, may be given at the candidate's place of employment or training by a qualified proctor
Examination format: Multiple choice and proficiency evaluation

Eligibility routes:	At least 6 months of full-time work experience in phlebotomy
	OR
	One year of part-time work experience in phlebotomy
	OR
	Completion of a formal training program that has been reviewed by the ASPT
Certification:	CPT (ASPT)
Recertification:	Certification must be renewed yearly by either re-examination or 6 contact hours per year of medically-related continuing education

The ASPT also certifies ECG Technicians, Paramedical Insurance Examiners, Point-of-Care Technicians, and Drug Collection Specialists.

5. *National Credentialing Agency for Medical Laboratory Personnel (NCA)*
8310 Nieman Road
Lenexa, KS 66214
Telephone: (913) 438-5110

Frequency of examination:	Twice per year; given only in designated cities
Examination format:	Multiple choice
Eligibility routes:	Completion of a formal education program
	OR
	One year of full-time work experience in phlebotomy
Certification:	CLPlb(NCA)
Recertification:	Recertification is every 2 years by 20 contact hours of continuing education or every 4 years by re-examination.

6. *National Phlebotomy Association (NPA)*
1901 Brightseat Road
Landover, MD 20785
Telephone: (301) 386-4200

Frequency of examination:	Varies with need; the NPA has a reclamation clause where experienced phlebotomists may be certified without examination.
Examination format:	Written portion and proficiency evaluation
Eligibility routes:	Working phlebotomist
	OR
	Completion of a phlebotomy training program
Certification:	CPT(NPA)
Recertification:	Recertification is yearly by 18 contact hours of continuing education

Index